RECENT TRENDS AND TECHNIQUES IN APPLIED GENETICS

RECENT TRENDS AND TECHNIQUES IN APPLIED GENETICS

Dr. R.N. Shukla

Oxford Book Company
Jaipur ▪ New Delhi

Published By

Oxford Book Company

Regd. Off. "Bony Residency", Gate No. 2
Opp. Tilak Public School, Vishweswariya Nagar,
Gopalpura Road, Jaipur - 302018, India
Ph: 0141 - 2761280, Telefax: 2761381
email - oxfordbookjpr@gmail.com
website - oxfordbookcompany.com

Delhi Office: 102, 1st Floor, Satyam House,
4327/3, Ansari Road, Darya Ganj,
New Delhi - 110002, India
Ph: 011-45652440

Distributed By
KEYA INTERNATIONAL PRESS LLP
E-mail: keyainternationalpressllp@gmail.com

Published in India, 2025

ISBN : 9789355240347

Typeset by Shivangi Computers, Jaipur

Printed and bound in India by Thomson Press Ltd.,
New Delhi

Contents

Preface

The most common form of genetic engineering involves the insertion of new genetic material at an unspecified location in the host genome. This is accomplished by isolating and copying the genetic material of interest, generating a construct containing all the genetic elements for correct expression, and then inserting this construct into the host organism. Other forms of genetic engineering include gene targeting and knocking out specific genes via engineered nucleases such as zinc finger nucleases or engineered homing endonucleases. Genetic engineering techniques have been applied in numerous fields including research, biotechnology, and medicine. Medicines such as insulin and human growth hormone are now produced in bacteria, experimental mice such as the oncomouse and the knockout mouse are being used for research purposes and insect resistant and/or herbicide tolerant crops have been commercialized. Genetically engineered plants and animals capable of producing biotechnology drugs more cheaply than current methods are also being developed and in 2009 the FDA approved the sale of the pharmaceutical protein antithrombin produced in the milk of genetically engineered goats.

The goal of functional genomics is to understand the relationship between an organism's genome and its phenotype. The term functional genomics is often used broadly to refer to the many possible approaches to understanding the properties and function of the entirety of an organism's genes and gene products. This definition is somewhat variable; Gibson and Muse define it as "approaches under development to ascertain the biochemical, cellular, and/or physiological properties of each and every gene product", while Pevsner includes the study of nongenic elements in his definition: "the genome-wide study of the function of DNA (including genes and nongenic elements), as well as the nucleic acid and protein products encoded by DNA". Because of its genome-wide approach, functional genomics requires the use of high-throughput technologies capable of assaying many functions or relationships simultaneously. Functional genomics involves studies of natural variation in genes, RNA, and proteins over time or space, as well as studies of natural or experimental functional disruptions affecting genes, chromosomes, RNAs, or proteins. The promise of functional genomics is to expand and synthesize genomic and proteomic knowledge into an understanding of the dynamic properties of an organism at cellular and/or organismal levels. This would provide a more complete picture of how biological function arises from the information encoded in an organism's genome. The possibility of understanding how a particular mutation leads to a given phenotype has important implications for human genetic diseases, as answering these questions could point scientists in the direction of a treatment or cure.

The book has been designed for university students and teachers dealing with genetics, molecular biology, genetic engineering and biochemistry.

— *Dr. R.N. Shukla*

Chapter 1

Human Genome Project

The Human Genome Project (HGP) is an international scientific research project with a primary goal of determining the sequence of chemical base pairs which make up DNA and to identify and map the approximately 20,000–25,000 genes of the human genome from both a physical and functional standpoint.

The project began in 1990 and was initially headed by [Ari Patrinos, head of the Office of Biological and Environmental Research. Francis Collins directed the National Institutes of Health National Human Genome Research Institute efforts]. A working draft of the genome was released in 2000 and a complete one in 2003, with further, more detailed analysis still being published. A parallel project was conducted outside of government by the Celera Corporation. Most of the government-sponsored sequencing was performed in universities and research centres from the United States, the United Kingdom, Japan, France, Germany and China. The mapping of human genes is an important step in the development of medicines and other aspects of health care.

While the objective of the Human Genome Project is to understand the genetic makeup of the human species, the project has also focused on several other nonhuman organisms such as *E. coli*, the fruit fly, and the laboratory mouse. It remains one of the largest single investigational projects in modern science.

The Human Genome Project originally aimed to map the nucleotides contained in a human haploid reference genome (more than three billion). Several groups have announced efforts to extend this to diploid human genomes including the International HapMap Project, Applied Biosystems, Perlegen, Illumina, JCVI, Personal Genome Project, and Roche-454.

The "genome" of any given individual (except for identical twins and cloned organisms) is unique; mapping "the human genome" involves sequencing multiple variations of each gene. The project did not study the entire DNA found in human cells; some heterochromatic areas (about 8% of the total genome) remain un-sequenced.

Project

The project began with the culmination of several years of work supported by the United States Department of Energy, in particular workshops in 1984 and 1986 and a subsequent initiative of the US Department of Energy. This 1987 report stated boldly, "The ultimate goal of this initiative is to understand the human genome" and "knowledge of the human as necessary to the continuing progress of medicine and other health sciences as knowledge of human anatomy has been for the present state of medicine." Candidate technologies were already being considered for the proposed undertaking at least as early as 1985.

James D. Watson was head of the National Centre for Human Genome Research at the National Institutes of Health (NIH) in the United States starting from 1988. Largely due to his disagreement with his boss, Bernadine Healy, over the issue of patenting genes, Watson was forced to resign in 1992. He was replaced by Francis Collins in April 1993, and the name of the Centre was changed to the National Human Genome Research Institute (NHGRI) in 1997.

The $3-billion project was formally founded in 1990 by the United States Department of Energy and the U.S. National Institutes of Health, and was expected to take 15 years. In addition to the United States, the international consortium comprised geneticists in the United Kingdom, France, Germany, Japan, China, and India.

Due to widespread international cooperation and advances in the field of genomics (especially in sequence analysis), as well as major advances in computing technology, a 'rough draft' of the genome was finished in 2000 (announced jointly by then US president Bill Clinton and the British Prime Minister Tony Blair on June 26, 2000). This first available rough draft assembly of the genome was completed by the UCSC Genome Bioinformatics Group, primarily led by then graduate student Jim Kent. Ongoing sequencing led to the announcement of the essentially complete genome in April 2003, 2 years earlier than planned. In May 2006, another milestone was passed on the way to completion of the project, when the sequence of the last chromosome was published in the journal Nature.

State of Completion

There are multiple definitions of the "complete sequence of the human genome". According to some of these definitions, the genome has already been completely sequenced, and according to other definitions, the genome has yet to be completely sequenced. There have been multiple popular press articles reporting that the genome was "complete." The genome has been completely sequenced using the definition employed by the International Human Genome Project. A graphical history of the human genome project shows that most of the human genome was complete by the end of 2003. However, there are a number of regions of the human genome that can be considered unfinished:

- First, the central regions of each chromosome, known as centromeres, are highly repetitive DNA sequences that are difficult to sequence using current technology. The centromeres are millions (possibly tens of millions) of base pairs long, and for the most part these are entirely un-sequenced.
- Second, the ends of the chromosomes, called telomeres, are also highly repetitive, and for most of the 46 chromosome ends these too are incomplete. It is not known precisely how much sequence remains before the telomeres of each chromosome are reached, but as with the centromeres, current technological restraints are prohibitive.
- Third, there are several loci in each individual's genome that contain members of multigene families that are difficult to disentangle with shotgun sequencing methods – these multigene families often encode proteins important for immune functions.
- Other than these regions, there remain a few dozen gaps scattered around the genome, some of them rather large, but there is hope that all these will be closed in the next couple of years.

In summary: the best estimates of total genome size indicate that about 92.3% of the genome has been completed and it is likely that the centromeres and telomeres will remain un-sequenced until new technology is developed that facilitates their sequencing. Most of the remaining DNA is highly repetitive and unlikely to contain genes, but it cannot be truly known until it is entirely sequenced. Understanding the functions of all the genes and their regulation is far from complete. The roles of junk DNA, the evolution of the genome, the differences between individuals, and many other questions are still the subject of intense interest by laboratories all over the world.

Goals

The sequence of the human DNA is stored in databases available to anyone on the Internet. The U.S. National Centre for Biotechnology Information (and sister organizations in Europe and Japan) house the gene sequence in a database known as GenBank, along with sequences of known and hypothetical genes and proteins. Other organizations such as the University of California, Santa Cruz, and Ensembl present additional data and annotation and powerful tools for visualizing and searching it. Computer programs have been developed to analyze the data, because the data itself is difficult to interpret without such programs.

The process of identifying the boundaries between genes and other features in a raw DNA sequence is called genome annotation and is the domain of bioinformatics. While expert biologists make the best annotators, their work proceeds slowly, and computer programs are increasingly used to meet the high-throughput demands of genome sequencing projects. The best current technologies for annotation make use of statistical models that take advantage of parallels between DNA sequences and human language, using concepts from computer science such as formal grammars.

Another, often overlooked, goal of the HGP is the study of its ethical, legal, and social implications. It is important to research these issues and find the most appropriate solutions before they become large dilemmas whose effect will manifest in the form of major political concerns.

All humans have unique gene sequences. Therefore the data published by the HGP does not represent the exact sequence of each and every individual's genome. It is the combined "reference genome" of a small number of anonymous donors. The HGP genome is a scaffold for future work in identifying differences among individuals. Most of the current effort in identifying differences among individuals involves single-nucleotide polymorphisms and the HapMap.

Findings

Key findings of the draft (2001) and complete (2004) genome sequences include

1. There are approximately 20,500 genes in human beings, the same range as in mice and twice that of roundworms. Understanding how these genes express themselves will provide clues to how diseases are caused.

2. Between 1.1% to 1.4% of the genome's sequence codes for proteins
3. The human genome has significantly more segmental duplications (nearly identical, repeated sections of DNA) than other mammalian genomes. These sections may underlie the creation of new primate-specific genes
4. At the time when the draft sequence was published less than 7% of protein families appeared to be vertebrate specific

How it was Accomplished

The Human Genome Project was started in 1989 with the goal of sequencing and identifying all three billion chemical units in the human genetic instruction set, finding the genetic roots of disease and then developing treatments. With the sequence in hand, the next step was to identify the genetic variants that increase the risk for common diseases like cancer and diabetes.

It was far too expensive at that time to think of sequencing patients' whole genomes. So the National Institutes of Health embraced the idea for a "shortcut", which was to look just at sites on the genome where many people have a variant DNA unit. The theory behind the shortcut was that since the major diseases are common, so too would be the genetic variants that caused them. Natural selection keeps the human genome free of variants that damage health before children are grown, the theory held, but fails against variants that strike later in life, allowing them to become quite common. (In 2002 the National Institutes of Health started a $138 million project called the HapMap to catalog the common variants in European, East Asian and African genomes.)

The genome was broken into smaller pieces; approximately 150,000 base pairs in length. These pieces were then ligated into a type of vector known as "bacterial artificial chromosomes", or BACs, which are derived from bacterial chromosomes which have been genetically engineered.

The vectors containing the genes can be inserted into bacteria where they are copied by the bacterial DNA replication machinery. Each of these pieces was then sequenced separately as a small "shotgun" project and then assembled. The larger, 150,000 base pairs go together to create chromosomes. This is known as the "hierarchical shotgun" approach, because the genome is first broken into relatively large chunks, which are then mapped to chromosomes before being selected for sequencing.

Funding came from the US government through the National Institutes of Health in the United States, and a UK charity organization, the Wellcome Trust, as well as numerous other groups from around the world. The funding supported a number of large sequencing centres including those at Whitehead Institute, the Sanger Centre, Washington University, and Baylor College of Medicine.

The Human Genome Project is considered a Mega Project because the human genome has approximately 3.3 billion base-pairs; if the cost of sequencing is US $3 per base-pair, then the approximate cost will be US $10 billion.

If the sequence obtained was to be stored in book form, and if each page contained 1000 base-pairs recorded and each book contained 1000 pages, then 3300 such books would be needed in order to store the complete genome. However, if expressed in units of computer data storage, 3.3 billion base-pairs recorded at 2 bits per pair would equal 786 megabytes of raw data. This is comparable to a fully data loaded CD.

Public Versus Private Approaches

In 1998, a similar, privately funded quest was launched by the American researcher Craig Venter, and his firm Celera Genomics. Venter was a scientist at the NIH during the early 1990s when the project was initiated. The $300,000,000 Celera effort was intended to proceed at a faster pace and at a fraction of the cost of the roughly $3 billion publicly funded project.

Celera used a technique called whole genome shotgun sequencing, employing pairwise end sequencing, which had been used to sequence bacterial genomes of up to six million base pairs in length, but not for anything nearly as large as the three billion base pair human genome.

Celera initially announced that it would seek patent protection on "only 200–300" genes, but later amended this to seeking "intellectual property protection" on "fully-characterized important structures" amounting to 100–300 targets. The firm eventually filed preliminary ("place-holder") patent applications on 6,500 whole or partial genes. Celera also promised to publish their findings in accordance with the terms of the 1996 "Bermuda Statement," by releasing new data annually (the HGP released its new data daily), although, unlike the publicly funded project, they would not permit free redistribution or scientific use of the data. The publicly funded competitor UC Santa Cruz was compelled to publish the first draft of the human genome before

Celera for this reason. On July 7, 2000, the UCSC Genome Bioinformatics Group released a first working draft on the web. The scientific community downloaded one-half trillion bytes of information from the UCSC genome server in the first 24 hours of free and unrestricted access to the first ever assembled blueprint of our human species. In March 2000, President Clinton announced that the genome sequence could not be patented, and should be made freely available to all researchers. The statement sent Celera's stock plummeting and dragged down the biotechnology-heavy Nasdaq. The biotechnology sector lost about $50 billion in market capitalization in two days.

Although the working draft was announced in June 2000, it was not until February 2001 that Celera and the HGP scientists published details of their drafts. Special issues of *Nature* (which published the publicly funded project's scientific paper) and *Science* (which published Celera's paper) described the methods used to produce the draft sequence and offered analysis of the sequence. These drafts covered about 83% of the genome (90% of the euchromatic regions with 150,000 gaps and the order and orientation of many segments not yet established). In February 2001, at the time of the joint publications, press releases announced that the project had been completed by both groups. Improved drafts were announced in 2003 and 2005, filling in to H"92% of the sequence currently.

The competition proved to be very good for the project, spurring the public groups to modify their strategy in order to accelerate progress. The rivals at UC Santa Cruz initially agreed to pool their data, but the agreement fell apart when Celera refused to deposit its data in the unrestricted public database GenBank. Celera had incorporated the public data into their genome, but forbade the public effort to use Celera data.

HGP is the most well known of many international genome projects aimed at sequencing the DNA of a specific organism. While the human DNA sequence offers the most tangible benefits, important developments in biology and medicine are predicted as a result of the sequencing of model organisms, including mice, fruit flies, zebrafish, yeast, nematodes, plants, and many microbial organisms and parasites.

In 2004, researchers from the International Human Genome Sequencing Consortium (IHGSC) of the HGP announced a new estimate of 20,000 to 25,000 genes in the human genome. Previously 30,000 to 40,000 had been predicted, while estimates at the start of the project reached up to as high as 2,000,000. The number continues to fluctuate and it is now expected that it will take many years to agree on a precise value for the number of genes in the human genome.

History

In 1976, the genome of the RNA virus Bacteriophage MS2 was the first complete genome to be determined, by Walter Fiers and his team at the University of Ghent (Ghent, Belgium). The idea for the shotgun technique came from the use of an algorithm that combined sequence information from many small fragments of DNA to reconstruct a genome. This technique was pioneered by Frederick Sanger to sequence the genome of the Phage Φ-X174, a virus (bacteriophage) that primarily infects bacteria that was the first fully sequenced genome (DNA-sequence) in 1977. The technique was called shotgun sequencing because the genome was broken into millions of pieces as if it had been blasted with a shotgun. In order to scale up the method, both the sequencing and genome assembly had to be automated, as they were in the 1980s.

It involved the use of automated sequencers, longer individual sequences using approximately 500 base pairs at that time. Paired sequences separated by a fixed distance of around 2000 base pairs which were critical elements enabling the development of the first genome assembly programs for reconstruction of large regions of genomes (aka 'contigs').

Three years later, in 1998, the announcement by the newly-formed Celera Genomics that it would scale up the pairwise end sequencing method to the human genome was greeted with skepticism in some circles. The shotgun technique breaks the DNA into fragments of various sizes, ranging from 2,000 to 300,000 base pairs in length, forming what is called a DNA "library". Using an automated DNA sequencer the DNA is read in 800bp lengths from both ends of each fragment. Using a complex genome assembly algorithm and a supercomputer, the pieces are combined and the genome can be reconstructed from the millions of short, 800 base pair fragments. The success of both the public and privately funded effort hinged upon a new, more highly automated capillary DNA sequencing machine, called the Applied Biosystems 3700, that ran the DNA sequences through an extremely fine capillary tube rather than a flat gel. Even more critical was the development of a new, larger-scale genome assembly program, which could handle the 30–50 million sequences that would be required to sequence the entire human genome with this method. At the time, such a program did not exist. One of the first major projects at Celera Genomics was the development of this assembler, which was written in parallel with the construction of a large, highly automated genome sequencing factory. Development of the assembler was led by Brian Ramos. The first version of this assembler was demonstrated in 2000, when the Celera team joined forces with Professor Gerald Rubin to sequence the fruit fly Drosophila melanogaster using the whole-genome shotgun method. At 130 million base pairs, it was at least 10 times larger than any genome previously shotgun assembled. One year later, the Celera team published their assembly of the three billion base pair human genome.

The Human Genome Project was a 13 year old mega project, that was launched in the year 1990 and completed in 2003. This project is closely associated to the branch of biology called Bio-informatics. The human genome project international consortium announced the publication of a draft sequence and analysis of the human genome—the genetic blueprint for the human being. An American company—Celera, led by Craig Venter and the other huge international collaboration of distinguished scientists led by Francis Collins, director, National Human Genome Research Institute, U.S., both published their findings. This Mega Project is co-ordinated by the U.S. Department of Energy and the National Institute of Health. During the early years of the project, the Wellcome Trust (U.K.) became a major partner, other countries like Japan, Germany, China and France contributed significantly. Already the atlas has revealed some starting facts. The two factors that made this project a success are:

1. Genetic Engineering Techniques, with which it is possible to isolate and clone any segment of DNA.
2. Availability of simple and fast technologies, to determining the DNA sequences.

Being the most complex organisms, human beings were expected to have more than 100,000 genes or combination of DNA that provides commands for every characteristics of the body. Instead their studies show that humans have only 30,000 genes – around the same as mice, three times as many as flies, and only five times more than bacteria. Scientist told that not only are the numbers similar, the genes themselves, baring a few, are alike in mice and men. In a companion volume to the Book of Life, scientists have created a catalogue of 1.4 million single-letter differences, or single-nucleotide polymorphisms (SNPs) – and specified their exact locations in the human genome. This SNP map, the world's largest publicly available catalogue of SNP's, promises to revolutionize both mapping diseases and tracing human history. The sequence information from the consortium has been immediately and freely released to the world, with no restrictions on its use or redistribution. The information is scanned daily by scientists in academia and industry, as well as commercial database companies, providing key information services to bio-technologists. Already, many genes have been identified from the genome sequence, including more than 30 that play a direct role in human diseases. By dating the three millions repeat elements and examining the pattern of interspersed repeats on the Y-chromosome, scientists estimated the relative mutation rates in the X and the Y chromosomes and in the male and the female germ lines. They found that the ratio of mutations in male Vs female is 2:1. Scientists point to several possible reasons for the higher mutation rate in the male germ line, including the fact that there are a greater number of cell divisions involved in the formation of sperm than in the formation of eggs.

Methods

The IHGSC used pair-end sequencing plus whole-genome shotgun mapping of large (H–100 Kbp) plasmid clones and shotgun sequencing of smaller plasmid sub-clones plus a variety of other mapping data to orient and check the assembly of each human chromosome.

The Celera group emphasized the importance of the "whole-genome shotgun" sequencing method, relying on sequence information to orient and locate their fragments within the chromosome. However they used the publicly available data from HGP to assist in the assembly and orientation process, raising concerns that the Celera sequence was not independently derived.

Genome Donors

In the IHGSC international public-sector Human Genome Project (HGP), researchers collected blood (female) or sperm (male) samples from a large number of donors. Only a few of many collected samples were processed as DNA resources. Thus the donor identities were protected so neither donors nor scientists could know whose DNA was sequenced. DNA clones from many different libraries were used in the overall project, with most of those libraries being created by Dr. Pieter J. de Jong. It has been informally reported, and is well known in the genomics community, that much of the DNA for the public HGP came from a single anonymous male donor from Buffalo, New York (code name RP11).

HGP scientists used white blood cells from the blood of two male and two female donors (randomly selected from 20 of each) — each donor yielding a separate DNA library. One of these libraries (RP11) was used considerably more than others, due to quality considerations. One minor technical issue is that male samples contain just over half as much DNA from the sex chromosomes (one X chromosome and one Y chromosome) compared to female samples (which contain two X chromosomes). The other 22 chromosomes (the autosomes) are the same for both genders.

Although the main sequencing phase of the HGP has been completed, studies of DNA variation continue in the International HapMap Project, whose goal is to identify patterns of single-nucleotide polymorphism (SNP) groups (called haplotypes, or "haps"). The DNA samples for the HapMap came from a total of 270 individuals: Yoruba people in Ibadan, Nigeria; Japanese people in Tokyo; Han Chinese in Beijing; and the French Centre d'Etude du Polymorphisms Humain (CEf) resource, which consisted of residents of the United States having ancestry from Western and Northern Europe.

In the Celera Genomics private-sector project, DNA from five different individuals were used for sequencing. The lead scientist of Celera Genomics at that time, Craig Venter, later acknowledged (in a public letter to the journal Science) that his DNA was one of 21 samples in the pool, five of which were selected for use.

On September 4, 2007, a team led by Craig Venter published his complete DNA sequence, unveiling the six-billion-nucleotide genome of a single individual for the first time.

Benefits

The work on interpretation of genome data is still in its initial stages. It is anticipated that detailed knowledge of the human genome will provide new avenues for advances in medicine and biotechnology. Clear practical results of the project emerged even before the work was finished. For example, a number of companies, such as Myriad Genetics started offering easy ways to administer genetic tests that can show predisposition to a variety of illnesses, including breast cancer, disorders of hemostasis, cystic fibrosis, liver diseases and many others. Also, the etiologies for cancers, Alzheimer's disease and other areas of clinical interest are considered likely to benefit from genome information and possibly may lead in the long term to significant advances in their management.

There are also many tangible benefits for biological scientists. For example, a researcher investigating a certain form of cancer may have narrowed down his/her search to a particular gene. By visiting the human genome database on the World Wide Web, this researcher can examine what other scientists have written about this gene, including (potentially) the three-dimensional structure of its product, its function(s), its evolutionary relationships to other human genes, or to genes in mice or yeast or fruit flies, possible detrimental mutations, interactions with other genes, body tissues in which this gene is activated, diseases associated with this gene or other datatypes.

Further, deeper understanding of the disease processes at the level of molecular biology may determine new therapeutic procedures. Given the established importance of DNA in molecular biology and its central role in determining the fundamental operation of cellular processes, it is likely that expanded knowledge in this area will facilitate medical advances in numerous areas of clinical interest that may not have been possible without them.

The analysis of similarities between DNA sequences from different organisms is also opening new avenues in the study of evolution. In many cases, evolutionary questions can now be framed in terms of molecular biology; indeed, many major evolutionary milestones (the emergence of the ribosome and organelles, the development of embryos with body plans, the vertebrate immune system) can be related to the molecular level. Many questions about the similarities and differences between humans and our closest relatives (the primates, and indeed the other mammals) are expected to be illuminated by the data from this project.

The Human Genome Diversity Project (HGDP), spinoff research aimed at mapping the DNA that varies between human ethnic groups, which was rumored to have been halted, actually did continue and to date has yielded new conclusions. In the future, HGDP could possibly expose new data in disease surveillance, human development and anthropology. HGDP could unlock secrets behind and create new strategies for managing the vulnerability of ethnic groups to certain diseases.

Advantages of Human Genome Project:

1. Knowledge of the effects of variation of DNA among individuals can revolutionize the ways to diagnose, treat and even prevent a number of diseases that affects the human beings.
2. It provides clues to the understanding of human biology.

Ethical, Legal and Social Issues

The project's goals included not only identifying all of the approximately 24,000 genes in the human genome, but also to address the ethical, legal, and social issues (ELSI) that might arise from the availability of genetic information. Five percent of the annual budget was allocated to address the ELSI arising from the project.

Debra Harry, Executive Director of the U.S group Indigenous Peoples Council on Biocolonialism (IPCB), says that despite a decade of ELSI funding, the burden of genetics education has fallen on the tribes themselves to understand the motives of Human genome project and its potential impacts on their lives. Meanwhile, the government has been busily funding projects studying indigenous groups without any meaningful consultation with the groups.

The main criticism of ELSI is the failure to address the conditions raised by population-based research, especially with regard to unique processes for group decision-making and cultural worldviews. Genetic variation research such as HGP is group population research, but most ethical guidelines, according to Harry, focus on individual rights instead of group rights. She says the research represents a clash of culture: indigenous people's life revolves around collectivity and group decision making whereas the Western culture promotes individuality. Harry suggests that one of the challenges of ethical research is to include respect for collective review and decision making, while also upholding the Western model of individual rights.

Cloning

Cloning in biology is the process of producing similar populations of genetically identical individuals that occurs in nature when organisms such as bacteria, insects or plants reproduce asexually. Cloning in biotechnology refers to processes used to create copies of DNA fragments (molecular cloning), cells (cell cloning), or organisms. The term also refers to the production of multiple copies of a product such as digital media or software.

Molecular Cloning

Molecular cloning refers to the process of making multiple molecules. Cloning is commonly used to amplify DNA fragments containing whole genes, but it can also be used to amplify any DNA sequence such as promoters, non-coding sequences and randomly fragmented DNA. It is used in a wide array of biological experiments and practical applications ranging from genetic fingerprinting to large scale protein production. Occasionally, the term cloning is misleadingly used to refer to the identification of the chromosomal location of a gene associated with a particular phenotype of interest, such as in positional cloning. In practice, localization of the gene to a chromosome or genomic region does not necessarily enable one to isolate or amplify the relevant genomic sequence. To amplify any DNA sequence in a living organism, that sequence must be linked to an origin of replication, which is a sequence of DNA capable of directing the propagation of itself and any linked sequence. However, a number of other features are needed and a variety of specialised cloning vectors (small piece of DNA into which a foreign DNA fragment can be inserted) exist that allow protein expression, tagging, single stranded RNA and DNA production and a host of other manipulations.

Cloning of any DNA fragment essentially involves four steps

1. fragmentation - breaking apart a strand of DNA
2. ligation - gluing together pieces of DNA in a desired sequence
3. transfection - inserting the newly formed pieces of DNA into cells
4. screening/selection - selecting out the cells that were successfully transfected with the new DNA.

Although these steps are invariable among cloning procedures a number of alternative routes can be selected, these are summarized as a 'cloning strategy'.

Initially, the DNA of interest needs to be isolated to provide a DNA segment of suitable size. Subsequently, a ligation procedure is used where the amplified fragment is inserted into a vector (piece of DNA). The vector (which is frequently circular) is linearised using restriction enzymes, and incubated with the fragment of interest under appropriate conditions with an enzyme called DNA ligase. Following ligation the vector with the insert of interest is transfected into cells. A number of alternative techniques are available, such as chemical sensitivation of cells, electroporation, optical injection and biolistics. Finally, the transfected cells are cultured. As the aforementioned procedures are of particularly low efficiency, there is a need to identify the cells that have been successfully transfected with the vector construct containing the desired insertion sequence in the required orientation. Modern cloning vectors include selectable antibiotic resistance markers, which allow only cells in which the vector has been transfected, to grow. Additionally, the cloning vectors may contain colour selection markers, which provide blue/white screening on X-gal medium. Nevertheless, these selection steps do not absolutely guarantee that the DNA insert is present in the cells obtained. Further investigation of the resulting colonies must be required to confirm that cloning was successful. This may be accomplished by means of PCR, restriction fragment analysis and/or DNA sequencing.

Unicellular Organisms

Cloning a cell means to derive a population of cells from a single cell. In the case of unicellular organisms such as bacteria and yeast, this process is remarkably simple and essentially only requires the inoculation of the appropriate medium. However, in the case of cell cultures from multi-cellular organisms, cell cloning is an arduous task as these cells will not readily grow in standard media.

A useful tissue culture technique used to clone distinct lineages of cell lines involves the use of cloning rings (cylinders). According to this technique, a single-cell suspension of cells that have been exposed to a mutagenic agent or drug used to drive selection is plated at high dilution to create isolated colonies; each arising from a single and potentially clonal distinct cell. At an early growth stage when colonies consist of only a few of cells, sterile polystyrene rings (cloning rings), which have been dipped in grease are placed over an individual colony and a small amount of trypsin is added. Cloned cells are collected from inside the ring and transferred to a new vessel for further growth.

Cloning in Stem Cell Research

Somatic cell nuclear transfer, known as SCNT, can also be used to create embryos for research or therapeutic purposes. The most likely purpose for this is to produce embryos for use in stem cell research. This process is also called "research cloning" or "therapeutic cloning." The goal is not to create cloned human beings (called "reproductive cloning"), but rather to harvest stem cells that can be used to study human development and to potentially treat disease. While a clonal human blastocyst has been created, stem cell lines are yet to be isolated from a clonal source.

Organism Cloning

Organism cloning (also called reproductive cloning) refers to the procedure of creating a new multicellular organism, genetically identical to another. In essence this form of cloning is an asexual method of reproduction, where fertilization or inter-gamete contact does not take place. Asexual reproduction is a naturally occurring phenomenon in many species, including most plants and some insects. Scientists have made some major achievements with cloning, including the asexual reproduction of sheep and cows. There is a lot of ethical debate over whether or not cloning should be used. However, cloning, or asexual propagation, has been common practice in the horticultural world for hundreds of years.

Horticultural

The term *clone* is used in horticulture to mean all descendants of a single plant, produced by vegetative reproduction or apomixis. Many horticultural plant cultivars are clones, having been derived from a single individual, multiplied by some process other than sexual reproduction. As an example, some European cultivars of grapes represent clones that have been propagated for over two millennia. Other examples are potato and banana. Grafting can be regarded as cloning, since all the shoots and branches coming from the graft are genetically a clone of a single individual, but this particular kind of cloning has not come under ethical scrutiny and is generally treated as an entirely different kind of operation.

Many trees, shrubs, vines, ferns and other herbaceous perennials form clonal colonies. Parts of a large clonal colony often become detached from the parent, termed fragmentation, to form separate individuals. Some plants also form seeds is asexually, termed apomixis, e.g. dandelion.

Parthenogenesis

Clonal derivation exists in nature in some animal species and is referred to as parthenogenesis (reproduction of an organism by itself without a mate). This is an asexual form of reproduction that is only found in females of some insects, crustaceans and lizards. The growth and development occurs without fertilization by a male. In plants, parthenogenesis means the development of an embryo from an unfertilized egg cell, and is a component process of apomixis. In species that use the XY sex-determination system, the offspring will always be female. An example is the "Little Fire Ant" (*Wasmannia auropunctata*), which is native to Central and South America but has spread throughout many tropical environments.

Artificial Cloning of Organisms

Artificial cloning of organisms may also be called *reproductive cloning.*

Methods

Reproductive cloning generally uses "somatic cell nuclear transfer" (SCNT) to create animals that are genetically identical. This process entails the transfer of a nucleus from a donor adult cell (somatic cell) to an egg that has no nucleus. If the egg begins to divide normally it is transferred into the uterus of the surrogate mother. Such clones are not strictly identical since the somatic cells may contain mutations in their nuclear DNA. Additionally, the mitochondria in the cytoplasm also contains DNA and during SCNT this DNA is wholly from the donor egg, thus the mitochondrial genome is not the same as that of the nucleus donor cell from which it was produced. This may have important implications for cross-species nuclear transfer in which nuclear-mitochondrial incompatibilities may lead to death.

Artificial *embryo splitting* or *embryo twinning* may also be used as a method of cloning, where an embryo is split in the maturation before embryo transfer. It is optimally performed at the 6- to 8-cell stage, where it can be used as an expansion of IVF to increase the number of available embryos. If both embryos are successful, it gives rise to monozygotic (identical) twins.

Dolly the Sheep

Dolly was publicly significant because the effort showed that the genetic material from a specific adult cell, programmed to express only a distinct subset of its genes, can be reprogrammed to grow an entirely new organism. Before this demonstration, it had been shown by John Gurdon that nuclei from differentiated cells could give rise to an entire organism after transplantation into an enucleated egg. However, this concept was not yet demonstrated in a mamallian system.

Cloning Dolly the sheep had a low success rate per fertilized egg; she was born after 237 eggs were used to create 29 embryos, which only produced three lambs at birth, only one of which lived. Seventy calves have been created and one third of them died young; Prometea took 277 attempts. Notably, although the first clones were frogs, no adult cloned frog has yet been produced from a somatic adult nucleus donor cell.

There were early claims that Dolly the Sheep had pathologies resembling accelerated aging. Scientists speculated that Dolly's death in 2003 was related to the shortening of telomeres, DNA-protein complexes that protect the end of linear chromosomes. However, other researchers, including Ian Wilmut who led the team that successfully cloned Dolly, argue that Dolly's early death due to respiratory infection was unrelated to deficiencies with the cloning process.

Species Cloned

The modern cloning techniques involving nuclear transfer have been successfully performed on several species. Landmark experiments in chronological order:

- Tadpole: (1952) Many scientists questioned whether cloning had actually occurred and unpublished experiments by other labs were not able to reproduce the reported results.
- Carp: (1963) In China, embryologist Tong Dizhou produced the world's first cloned fish by inserting the DNA from a cell of a male carp into an egg from a female carp. He published the findings in a Chinese science journal.
- Mice: (1986) A mouse was the first mammal successfully cloned from an early embryonic cell. Soviet scientists Chaylakhyan, Veprencev, Sviridova, and Nikitin had the mouse "Masha" cloned. Research was published in the magazine "Biofizika" volume ÕÕÕII, issue 5 of 1987.
- Sheep: (1996) From early embryonic cells by Steen Willadsen. Megan and Morag cloned from differentiated embryonic cells in June 1995 and Dolly the sheep from a somatic cell in 1997.
- Rhesus Monkey: Tetra (January 2000) from embryo splitting
- Gaur: (2001) was the first endangered species cloned.
- Cattle: Alpha and Beta (males, 2001) and (2005) Brazil
- Cat: CopyCat "CC" (female, late 2001), Little Nicky, 2004, was the first cat cloned for commercial reasons
- Dog: Snuppy, a male Afghan hound was the first cloned dog (2005).
- Rat: Ralph, the first cloned rat (2003)
- Mule: Idaho Gem, a john mule born 4 May 2003, was the first horse-family clone.
- Horse: Prometea, a Haflinger female born 28 May 2003, was the first horse clone.
- Water Buffalo: Samrupa was the first cloned water buffalo. It was born on February 6, 2009, at India's Karnal National Diary Research Institute but died five days later due to lung infection.
- Camel: (2009) Injaz, is the first cloned camel.

Human Cloning

Human cloning is the creation of a genetically identical copy of an existing or previously existing human. The term is generally used to refer to *artificial* human cloning; human clones in the form of identical twins are commonplace, with their cloning occurring during the natural process of reproduction. There are two commonly discussed types of human cloning: therapeutic cloning and reproductive cloning. Therapeutic cloning involves cloning adult cells for use in medicine and is an active area of research. Reproductive cloning would involve making cloned humans. A third type of cloning called replacement cloning is a theoretical possibility, and would be a combination of therapeutic and reproductive cloning. Replacement cloning would entail the replacement of an extensively damaged, failed, or failing body through cloning followed by whole or partial brain transplant.

The various forms of human cloning are controversial. There have been numerous demands for all progress in the human cloning field to be halted. Most scientific, governmental and religious organizations oppose reproductive cloning. The American Association for the Advancement of Science (AAAS) and other scientific organizations have made public statements suggesting that human reproductive cloning be banned until safety issues are resolved. Serious ethical concerns have been raised by the future possibility of harvesting organs from clones. Some people have considered the idea of growing organs separately from a human organism - in doing this, a new organ supply could be established without the moral implications of harvesting them from humans. Research is also being done on the idea of growing organs that are biologically acceptable to the human body inside of other organisms, such as pigs or cows, then transplanting them to humans, a form of xenotransplantation.

The first human hybrid human clone was created in November 1998, by American Cell Technologies. It was created from a man's leg cell, and a cow's egg whose DNA was removed. It was destroyed after 12 days. Since a normal embryo implants at 14 days, Dr Robert Lanza, ACT's director of tissue engineering, told the Daily Mail newspaper that the embryo could not be seen as a person before 14 days. While making an embryo, which may have resulted in a complete human had it been allowed to come to term, according to ACT: "[ACT's] aim was 'therapeutic cloning' not 'reproductive cloning'"

On January, 2008, Wood and Andrew French, Stemagen's chief scientific officer in California, announced that they successfully created the first 5 mature human embryos using DNA from adult skin cells, aiming to provide a source of viable embryonic stem cells. Dr. Samuel Wood and a colleague donated skin cells, and DNA from those cells was transferred to human eggs. It is not clear if the embryos produced would have been capable of further development, but Dr. Wood stated that if that were possible, using the technology for reproductive cloning would be both unethical and illegal. The 5 cloned embryos, created in Stemagen Corporation lab, in La Jolla, were destroyed.

Ethical Issues of Cloning

Because of recent technological advancements, the cloning of animals (and potentially humans) has been an issue. The Catholic Church and many religious organizations oppose all forms of cloning, on the grounds that life begins at conception. Judaism does not equate life with conception and, though some question the wisdom of cloning, Orthodox rabbis generally find no firm reason in Jewish law and ethics to object to cloning. From the standpoint of classical liberalism, concerns also exist regarding the protection of the identity of the individual and the right to protect one's genetic identity.

Gregory Stock is a scientist and outspoken critic against restrictions on cloning research. Bioethicist Gregory Pence also attacks the idea of criminalizing attempts to clone humans. The social implications of an artificial human production scheme were famously explored in Aldous Huxley's novel *Brave New World.*

On December 28, 2006, the U.S. Food and Drug Administration (FDA) approved the consumption of meat and other products from cloned animals. Cloned-animal products were said to be virtually indistinguishable from the non-cloned animals. Furthermore, companies would not be required to provide labels informing the consumer that the meat comes from a cloned animal.

Critics have raised objections to the FDA's approval of cloned-animal products for human consumption, arguing that the FDA's research was inadequate, inappropriately limited, and of questionable scientific validity. Several consumer-advocate groups are working to encourage a tracking program that would allow consumers to become more aware of cloned-animal products within their food.

Joseph Mendelson, legal director of the Centre for Food Safety, said that cloned food still should be labelled since safety and ethical issues about it remain questionable. Carol Tucker Foreman, director of food policy at the Consumer Federation of America, stated that FDA does not consider the fact that the results of some studies revealed that cloned animals have increased rates of mortality and deformity at birth.

Cloning Extinct and Endangered Species

Cloning, or more precisely, the reconstruction of functional DNA from extinct species has, for decades, been a dream of some scientists. The possible implications of this were dramatized in the best-selling novel by Michael Crichton and high budget Hollywood thriller *Jurassic Park.* In real life, one of the most anticipated targets for cloning was once the Woolly Mammoth, but attempts to extract DNA from frozen mammoths have been unsuccessful, though a joint Russo-Japanese team is currently working toward this goal.

In 2001, a cow named Bessie gave birth to a cloned Asian gaur, an endangered species, but the calf died after two days. In 2003, a banteng was successfully cloned, followed by three African wildcats from a thawed frozen embryo. These successes provided hope that similar techniques (using surrogate mothers of another species) might be used to clone extinct species. Anticipating this possibility, tissue samples from the last *bucardo* (Pyrenean Ibex) were frozen in liquid nitrogen immediately after it died in 2000. Researchers are also considering cloning endangered species such as the giant panda, ocelot, and cheetah. The "Frozen Zoo" at the San Diego Zoo now stores frozen tissue from the world's rarest and most endangered species.

In 2002, geneticists at the Australian Museum announced that they had replicated DNA of the Thylacine (Tasmanian Tiger), extinct about 65 years previous, using polymerase chain reaction. However, on February 15, 2005 the museum announced that it was stopping the project after tests showed the specimens' DNA had been too badly degraded by the (ethanol) preservative. On 15 May 2005 it was announced that the Thylacine project would be revived, with new participation from researchers in New South Wales and Victoria. In January 2009, for the first time, an extinct animal, the Pyrenean ibex mentioned above was cloned, at the Centre of Food Technology and Research of Aragon, using the preserved DNA of the skin samples from 2001 and domestic goat egg-cells. (The ibex died shortly after birth due to physical defects in its lungs.) One of the continuing obstacles in the attempt to clone extinct species is the need for nearly perfect DNA. Cloning from a single specimen could not create a viable breeding population in sexually reproducing animals. Furthermore, even if males and females were to be cloned, the question would remain open whether they would be viable at all in the absence of parents that could teach or show them their natural behaviour.

Cloning endangered species is a highly ideological issue. Many conservation biologists and environmentalists vehemently oppose cloning endangered species — mainly because they think it may deter donations to help preserve natural habitat and wild animal populations. The "rule-of-thumb" in animal conservation is that, if it is still feasible to conserve habitat and viable wild populations, breeding in captivity should not be undertaken in isolation.

Chapter 2

Functional Genomics

Functional genomics is a field of molecular biology that attempts to make use of the vast wealth of data produced by genomic projects (such as genome sequencing projects) to describe gene (and protein) functions and interactions. Unlike genomics and proteomics, functional genomics focuses on the dynamic aspects such as gene transcription, translation, and protein-protein interactions.

Goals of Functional Genomics

The goal of functional genomics is to understand the relationship between an organism's genome and its phenotype. The term functional genomics is often used broadly to refer to the many possible approaches to understanding the properties and function of the entirety of an organism's genes and gene products. This definition is somewhat variable; Gibson and Muse define it as "approaches under development to ascertain the biochemical, cellular, and/or physiological properties of each and every gene product", while Pevsner includes the study of nongenic elements in his definition: "the genome-wide study of the function of DNA (including genes and nongenic elements), as well as the nucleic acid and protein products encoded by DNA". Because of its genome-wide approach, functional genomics requires the use of high-throughput technologies capable of assaying many functions or relationships simultaneously. Functional genomics involves studies of natural variation in genes, RNA, and proteins over time (such as an organism's development) or space (such as its body regions), as well as studies of natural or experimental functional disruptions affecting genes, chromosomes, RNAs, or proteins.

The promise of functional genomics is to expand and synthesize genomic and proteomic knowledge into an understanding of the dynamic properties of an organism at cellular and/or organismal levels. This would provide a more complete picture of how biological function arises from the information encoded in an organism's genome.

The possibility of understanding how a particular mutation leads to a given phenotype has important implications for human genetic diseases, as answering these questions could point scientists in the direction of a treatment or cure.

Techniques and Applications

Functional genomics includes function-related aspects of the genome itself such as mutation and polymorphism (such as SNP) analysis, as well as measurement of molecular activities. The latter comprise a number of "-omics" such as transcriptomics (gene expression), proteomics (protein expression), phosphoproteomics (a subset of proteomics) and metabolomics. Functional genomics uses mostly multiplex techniques to measure the abundance of many or all gene products such as mRNAs or proteins within a biological sample. Together these measurement modalities endeavor to quantitate the various biological processes and improve our understanding of gene and protein functions and interactions.

At the DNA Level

Genetic Interaction Mapping

Systematic pairwise deletion of genes or inhibition of gene expression can be used to identify genes with related function, even if they do not interact physically. Epistasis refers to the fact that effects for two different gene knockouts may not be additive; that is, the phenotype that results when two genes are inhibited may be different from the sum of the effects of single knockouts.

The ENCODE Project

The ENCODE (Encyclopedia of DNA elements) project is an in-depth analysis of the human genome whose goal is to identify all the functional elements of genomic DNA, in both coding and noncoding regions. To this point, only the pilot phase of the study has been completed, involving hundreds of assays performed on 44 regions of known or unknown function comprising 1% of the human genome. Important results include evidence from genomic tiling arrays that most nucleotides are transcribed as coding transcripts, noncoding RNAs, or random transcripts, the discovery of additional transcriptional regulatory sites, further elucidation of chromatin-modifying mechanisms.

At the RNA Level: Transcriptome Profiling

Microarrays

Microarrays measure the amount of mRNA in a sample that corresponds to a given gene or probe DNA sequence. Probe sequences are immobilized on a solid surface and allowed to hybridize with fluorescently-labelled "target" mRNA. The intensity of fluorescence of a spot is proportional to the amount of target sequence that has hybridized to that spot, and therefore to the abundance of that mRNA sequence in the sample. Microarrays allow for identification of candidate genes involved in a given process based on variation between transcript levels for different conditions and shared expression patterns with genes of known function.

SAGE

SAGE (Serial analysis of gene expression) is an alternate method of gene expression analysis based on RNA sequencing rather than hybridization. SAGE relies on the sequencing of 10-17 base pair tags which are unique to each gene. These tags are produced from poly-A mRNA and ligated end-to-end before sequencing. SAGE gives an unbiased measurement of the number of transcripts per cell, since it does not depend on prior knowledge of what transcripts to study (as microarrays do).

At the Protein Level: Protein-protein Interactions

Yeast two-hybrid System

A yeast two-hybrid (Y2H) screen tests a "bait" protein against many potential interacting proteins ("prey") to identify physical protein-protein interactions. This system is based on a transcription factor, originally GAL4, whose separate DNA-binding and transcription activation domains are both required in order for the protein to cause transcription of a reporter gene. In a Y2H screen, the "bait" protein is fused to the binding domain of GAL4, and a library of potential "prey" (interacting) proteins is recombinantly expressed in a vector with the activation domain. In vivo interaction of bait and prey proteins in a yeast cell brings the activation and binding domains of GAL4 close enough together to result in expression of a reporter gene.

It is also possible to systematically test a library of bait proteins against a library of prey proteins to identify all possible interactions in a cell.

AP/MS

Affinity purification and mass spectrometry (AP/MS) is able to identify proteins that interact with one another in complexes. Complexes of proteins are allowed to form around a particular "bait" protein. The bait protein is identified using an antibody or a recombinant tag which allows it to be extracted along with any proteins that have formed a complex with it. The proteins are then digested into short peptide fragments and mass spectrometry is used to identify the proteins based on the mass-to-charge ratios of those fragments.

Loss-of-function Techniques

Mutagenesis

Gene function can be investigated by systematically "knocking out" genes one by one. This is done by either deletion or disruption of function (such as by insertional mutagenesis) and the resulting organisms are screened for phenotypes that provide clues to the function of the disrupted gene.

RNAi

RNA interference (RNAi) methods can be used to transiently silence or knock down gene expression using ~20 base-pair double-stranded RNA typically delivered by transfection of synthetic ~20-mer short-interfering RNA molecules (siRNAs) or by virally-encoded short-hairpin RNAs (shRNAs). RNAi screens, typically performed in cell culture-based assays or experimental organisms (such as C. elegans) can be used to systematically disrupt nearly every gene in a genome or subsets of genes (sub-genomes); possible functions of disrupted genes can be assigned based on observed phenotypes.

Functional Annotations for Genes

Genome Annotation

Putative genes can be identified by scanning a genome for regions likely to encode proteins, based on characteristics such as long open reading frames, transcriptional initiation sequences, and polyadenylation sites.

A sequence identified as a putative gene must be confirmed by further evidence, such as similarity to cDNA or EST sequences from the same organism, similarity of the predicted protein sequence to known proteins, association with promoter sequences, or evidence that mutating the sequence produces an observable phenotype.

Rosetta Stone Approach

The Rosetta stone approach is a computation method of de novo protein function prediction, based on the hypothesis that some proteins involved in a given physiological process may exist as two separate genes in one organism and as a single gene in another. Genomes are scanned for sequences that are independent in one organism and in a single open reading frame in another. If two genes have fused, it is predicted that they have similar biological functions that make such coregulation advantageous.

Functional Genomics and Bioinformatics

Because of the large quantity of data produced by these techniques and the desire to find biologically meaningful patterns, bioinformatics is crucial to analysis of functional genomics data. Examples of techniques in this class are data clustering or principal component analysis for unsupervised machine learning (class detection) as well as artificial neural networks or support vector machines for supervised machine learning (class prediction, classification).

Structural Genomics

Structural genomics seeks to describe the 3-dimensional structure of every protein encoded by a given genome. This genome-based approach allows for a high-throughput method of structure determination by a combination of experimental and modeling approaches.

The principle difference between structural genomics and traditional structural prediction is that structural genomics attempts to determine the structure of every protein encoded by the genome, rather than focusing on one particular protein. What is it that makes it possible to determine the structure of every protein in the genome at once rather than solve the structures one at a time? With full-genome sequences available, structure prediction can be done more quickly through a combination of experimental and modeling approaches, especially because the availability of large number of sequenced genomes and previously-solved protein structures allows scientists to model protein structure on the structures of previously solved homologs.

Because protein structure is closely linked with protein function, the structural genomics has the potential to inform knowledge of protein function. In addition to elucidating protein functions, structural genomics can be used to identify novel protein folds and potential targets for drug discovery. Structural genomics involves taking a large number of approaches to structure determination, including experimental methods using genomic sequences or modeling-based approaches based on sequence or structural homology to a protein of known structure or based on chemical and physical principles for a protein with no homology to any known structure.

As opposed to traditional structural biology, the determination of a protein structure through a structural genomics effort often (but not always) comes before anything is known regarding the protein function. This raises new challenges in structural bioinformatics, i.e. determining protein function from its 3D structure.

Structural genomics emphasizes high throughput determination of protein structures. This is performed in dedicated centres of structural genomics.

While most structural biologists pursue structures of individual proteins or protein groups, specialists in structural genomics pursue structures of proteins on a genome wide scale. This implies large scale cloning, expression and purification. One main advantage of this approach is economy of scale. On the other hand, the scientific value of some resultant structures is at times questioned. A *Science* article from January 2006 analyzes the structural genomics field.

One advantage of structural genomics, such as the Protein Structure Initiative, is that the scientific community gets immediate access to new structures, as well as to reagents such as clones and protein. A disadvantage is that many of these structures are of proteins of unknown function and do not have corresponding publications. This requires new ways of communicating this structural information to the broader research community. The Bioinformatics core of the Joint centre for structural genomics (JCSG) has recently developed a wiki-based approach namely The Open Protein Structure Annotation Network (TOPSAN) for annotating protein structures emerging from high-throughput structural genomics centres.

Goals

One goal of structural genomics is to identify novel protein folds. Experimental methods of protein structure determination require proteins that express and/or crystallize well, which may inherently bias the kinds of proteins folds that this experimental data elucidate. A genomic, modeling-based approach such as *ab initio* modeling may be better able to identify novel protein folds than the experimental approaches because they are not limited by experimental constraints.

Protein function depends on 3-D structure and these 3-D structures are more highly-conserved than sequences. Thus, the high-throughput structure determination methods of structural genomics have the potential to inform our understanding of protein functions. This also has potential implications for drug discovery and protein engineering. Furthermore, every protein that is added to the structural database increases the likelihood that the database will include homologous sequences of other unknown proteins. The Protein Structure Initiative (PSI) is a multifaceted effort funded by the National Institutes of Health with various academic and industrial partners that aims to increase knowledge of protein structure using a structural genomics approach and to improve structure-determination methodology.

Methods

Structural genomics takes advantage of completed genome sequences in several ways in order to determine protein structures. The gene sequence of the target protein can also be compared to a known sequence and structural information can then be inferred from the known protein's structure. Structural genomics can be used to predict novel protein folds based on other structural data. Structural genomics can also take modeling-based approach that relies on homology between the unknown protein and a solved protein structure.

De Novo Methods

Completed genome sequences allow every open reading frame (ORF), the part of a gene that is likely to contain the sequence for the mRNA and protein, to be cloned and expressed as protein. These proteins are then purified and crystallized, and then subjected to one of two types of structure determination: X-ray crystallography and [Nuclear Magnetic Resonance (NMR). The whole genome sequence allows for the design of every primer required in order to amplify all of the ORFs, clone them into bacteria, and then express them. By using a whole-genome approach to this traditional method of protein structure determination, all of the proteins encoded by the genome can be expressed at once. This approach allows for the structural determination of every protein that is encoded by the genome.

Modelling-based Methods

Ab Initio Modeling

This approach uses protein sequence data and the chemical and physical interactions of the encoded amino acids to predict the 3-D structures of proteins with no homology to solved protein structures.

One highly successful method for *ab initio* modeling is the Rosetta program, which divides the protein into short segments and arranges short polypeptide chain into a low-energy local conformation. Rosetta is available for commercial use and for non-commercial use through its public program, Robetta.

Sequence-based Modeling

This modeling technique compares the gene sequence of an unknown protein with sequences of proteins with known structures. Depending on the degree of similarity between the sequences, the structure of the known protein can be used as a model for solving the structure of the unknown protein. Highly accurate modeling is considered to require at least 50% amino acid sequence identity between the unknown protein and the solved structure. 30-50% sequence identity gives a model of intermediate-accuracy, and sequence identity below 30% gives low-accuracy models. It has been predicted that at least 16,000 protein structures will need to be determined in order for all structural motifs to be represented at least once and thus allowing the structure of any unknown protein to be solved accurately through modeling. One disadvantage of this method, however, is that structure is more conserved than sequence and thus sequence-based modeling may not be the most accurate way to predict protein structures.

Threading

Threading bases structural modeling on fold similarities rather than sequence identity. This method may help identify distantly-related proteins and can be used to infer molecular functions.

Examples of Structural Genomics

There are currently a number of on-going efforts to solve the structures for every protein in a given proteome.

The Thermotogo Maritima Proteome

One current goal of the Joint Centre for Structural Genomics (JCSG), a part of the Protein Structure Initiative (PSI) is to solve the structures for all the proteins in *Thermotogo maritima*, a thermophillic bacterium. *T. maritima* was selected as a structural genomics target based on its relatively small genome consisting of 1,877 genes and the hypothesis that the proteins expressed by a thermophilic bacterium would be easier to crystallize.

Lesley *et al* used *Escherichia coli* to express all the open-reading frames (ORFs) of *T. martima*. These proteins were then crystallized and structures were determined for successfully-crystallized proteins using X-ray crystallography. Among other structures, this structural genomics approach allowed for the determination of the structure of the TM0449 protein, which was found to exhibit a novel fold as it did not share structural homology with any known protein.

The Mycobacterium Tuberculosis Proteome

The goal of the TB Structural Genomics Consortium is to determine the structures of potential drug targets in *Mycobacterium tuberculosis*, the bacterium that causes tuberculosis. The development of novel drug therapies against tuberculosis are particularly important given the growing problem of multi-drug-resistant tuberculosis. The fully sequenced genome of *M. tuberculosis* has allowed scientists to clone many of these protein targets into expression vectors for purification and structure determination by X-ray crystallography. Studies have identified a number of target proteins for structure determination, including extracellular proteins that may be involved in pathogenesis, iron-regulatory proteins, current drug targets, and proteins predicted to have novel folds. So far, structures have been determined for 708 of the proteins encoded by *M. tuberculosis*.

Protein Structure Databases and Classifications

Protein Data Bank (PDB): repository for protein sequence and structural information. UniProt: provides sequence and functional information. Structural Classification of Proteins (SCOP Classifications): hierarchical-based approach Class, Architecture, Topology and Homologous superfamily (CATH): hierarchical-based approach.

Comparative Genomics

Comparative genomics is the study of the relationship of genome structure and function across different biological species or strains. Comparative genomics is an attempt to take advantage of the information provided by the signatures of selection to understand the function and evolutionary processes that act on genomes. While it is still a young field, it holds great promise to yield insights into many aspects of the evolution of modern species. The sheer amount of information contained in modern genomes (3.2 gigabases in the case of humans) necessitates that the methods of comparative genomics are automated. Gene finding is an important application of comparative genomics, as is discovery of new, non-coding functional elements of the genome.

Comparative genomics exploits both similarities and differences in the proteins, RNA, and regulatory regions of different organisms to infer how selection has acted upon these elements. Those elements that are responsible for similarities between different species should be conserved through time (stabilizing selection), while those elements responsible for differences among species should be divergent (positive selection). Finally, those elements that are unimportant to the evolutionary success of the organism will be unconserved (selection is neutral).

One of the important goals of the field is the identification of the mechanisms of eukaryotic genome evolution. It is however often complicated by the multiplicity of events that have taken place throughout the history of individual lineages, leaving only distorted and superimposed traces in the genome of each living organism. For this reason comparative genomics studies of small model organisms (for example yeast) are of great importance to advance our understanding of general mechanisms of evolution.

Having come a long way from its initial use of finding functional proteins, comparative genomics is now concentrating on finding regulatory regions and siRNA molecules. Recently, it has been discovered that distantly related species often share long conserved stretches of DNA that do not appear to code for any protein. One such ultra-conserved region, that was stable from chicken to chimp has undergone a sudden burst of change in the human lineage, and is found to be active in the developing brain of the human embryo.

Computational approaches to genome comparison have recently become a common research topic in computer science. A public collection of case studies and demonstrations is growing, ranging from whole genome comparisons to gene expression analysis. This has increased the introduction of different ideas, including concepts from systems and control, information theory, strings analysis and data mining. It is anticipated that computational approaches will become and remain a standard topic for research and teaching, while multiple courses will begin training students to be fluent in both topics.

Genomics for Health Improvement

Over the last 100 years, innovations in science and technology, together with improved socio-economic conditions, have resulted in improved health, quality of life and a vast increase in people's life expectancy worldwide. In light of this impressive record it is disheartening that the benefits of modern medicine still do not reach billions of people in the poorer parts of the world. Children and adults are undernourished, live in poor housing with few modern facilities, such as clean, running water, and die from various, often preventable, illnesses in the prime of their lives.

While there are many factors that come into play in the complex issue of development, it is widely accepted that science and technology plays a critical role in improving health in developing countries. Genomics and related biotechnologies constitute an exciting new field of science that possesses tremendous potential to address health problems in developing countries – if we rise to the challenge.

The purpose of this report is to focus on the role of genomics and related health biotechnologies as an example of the application of science, technology and innovation (STI) to improve global health and contribute towards meeting the United Nations Millennium Development Goals. The Millennium Development Goals (MDGs) grew out of the commitment of the United Nations to promote sustained development and eliminate poverty all over the world. They help quantify progress by defining targets and indicators to measure them. The first seven MDGs are directed at specific objectives in promoting development and improving people's lives, while the eighth goal, 'a global partnership for development', focuses on the means to achieve them. Many of the goals address health issues directly, such as improving infant and maternal health and reducing the prevalence of infectious diseases. The MDGs have become the international standard for measuring and tracking improvements in development. Therefore, the MDGs have the advantage of (i) agreement and support with the leaders of all UN member states, (ii) offering a comprehensive and multi-dimensional development framework, and (iii) setting clear quantifiable goals for all countries to meet by 2015. Although the MDGs, especially the health-related ones, have their critics, they do represent a standard by which progress may be measured.

The Millennium Project, whose mission is to devise and recommend operational frameworks to help developing countries achieve the MDGs, has set up ten thematically oriented task forces, consisting of experts and leading practitioners. These task forces have carried out detailed and comprehensive research in each thematic area on the science, public health needs and medical interventions, as well as the social, political and economic issues. The goals of the Science and Technology Task Force are to address how science and technology can be enhanced and applied to help all countries achieve the MDGs. Its mission is guided by the understanding that most of the MDGs cannot be reached without a strong contribution from science and technology.

The Potential of Genomics

Medicine and the biomedical sciences are currently in the midst of a fundamental change that is fuelled by the genomics revolution. In its report on "Genomics and World Health" the World Health Organization's Advisory Committee on Health Research observed that the application of knowledge gained from the characterization of the genomes of organisms holds enormous potential for the development of new health care innovations over the coming decades. With increased understanding of the molecular basis of diseases and their causation, the way we identify, prevent, diagnose, and treat diseases in the new millennium is bound to change.

The science of genomics is generating vast amounts of new knowledge. Once generated, this knowledge can be used creatively in the development of new diagnostic technologies, treatments and preventive programs.

Genomics requires massive amounts of information to be collected and analysed. The field has evolved over the last few decades in large part due to advances in sequencing technology, as well as information and communication technology. Automated DNA sequencing and genotyping have made it possible to characterize rapidly large numbers of genes. The means to manage, store and process enormous databases of biological information have spawned an entirely new field – bioinformatics.

These developments hold tremendous promise for the prevention, diagnosis and treatment of some of the major diseases affecting humankind, including HIV, malaria, and tuberculosis, as well as non-communicable diseases such as diabetes, cancer and cardiovascular disease. Genomics can also be applied to understand the genetics of bacteria, plants, and animals. Many genomes have been sequenced and mapped. In fact, the first genome sequence (that of *H. influenzae*) was completed in 1995, by researchers at The Institute for Genomic Research (TIGR). The sequence was a mere 1.8 million base-pairs, compared with the 3.2 billion base-pairs of the human genome. Many other genomes of the plant and animal kingdom have been sequenced, ranging from common yeast to rice, and all these sequencing achievements promise to enhance scientific knowledge. In October 2002, scientists published the sequence of the parasites responsible for human malaria, *Plasmodium falciparum*, as well as the mosquito that carries it, *Anopheles gambiae*. The knowledge of these genomes, together with the knowledge of the human genome, can be used to develop new drug and vaccine targets against malaria.

There may also be direct *economic* benefits of genomics. It is already a significant contributor to the biotechnology sector. Despite early setbacks, the genomics-based pharmaceutical market was expected to grow from US $2.2 billion in 1999 to US $8.2 billion in 2004. The major economic players in the world are not the only ones expected to benefit from genomics. Cuba, for example, has invested heavily since the 1980's in research infrastructure and manufacturing in biotechnology. As a result biotechnology is poised to become a major export industry in Cuba. In order to reap direct economic benefit from genomics, countries will have to be active participants in the development and manufacturing of genomics products. Those countries that will benefit the most from genomics are those that have appropriate health products to improve the health of their populations and who are active in developing and supplying those products. This will involve engaging and stimulating the private sector, without which the production and commercialization of new biotechnology products will be a challenge. As highlighted by the UN Commission on Private Sector and Development report, "*Unleashing Entrepreneurship: Making Business Work for the Poor*," the process of commercialization for development involves the dissemination and facilitation of knowledge flows between public and private sectors of both developed and developing markets. The report recommends action in both the public and private spheres, but also emphasizes the linkages between these spheres, recognizing the importance of cooperation and partnerships to achieve goals.

Molecular Diagnostics

- Combat HIV/AIDS, malaria and other diseases
- Reduce child mortality
- Improve maternal health.

Molecular diagnostics draw upon recent advances in biology to diagnose infectious disease by detecting the presence or absence of pathogen-associated molecules, such as DNA or protein, in a patient's blood or tissues. They present a powerful set of methods to address the health-related Millennium Development Goals, *Combat HIV/ AIDS,* malaria and other diseases, Reduce child mortality, Improve *maternal health.* Infectious and parasitic diseases are responsible for nearly 40%, or 17 million of all deaths every year. The three major killers are HIV/AIDS, malaria and tuberculosis, which together claim at least 5 million lives a year. Each year an estimated 11 million children still die before reaching their fifth birthday.

While improving public health infrastructure for disease prevention is crucial to the achievement of this goal, it is also true that once disease strikes, diagnosis and treatment methods are essential. Rapid and accurate diagnosis not only increases chances of survival, but also avoids waste of resources on inappropriate treatments and helps contain disease. It is not surprising that the scientific panel in the University of Toronto study ranked molecular diagnostics as the most promising set of technologies for improving health in developing countries over the next five to ten years. Many of the diagnostic tools currently in use in developing countries are cumbersome, time-consuming and expensive. In contrast, molecular diagnostics are simple to use, give quick results and can be relatively cheap. We focus on a few such technologies: polymerase chain reaction, monoclonal antibodies and recombinant antigens.

The *polymerase chain reaction* (PCR) is a quick way of making millions of copies of a specific sequence of DNA. This technology is fast and accurate. It takes advantage of the fact that organisms have unique genetic sequences. Amplification and identification of a pathogen-specific DNA sequence in the body fluids or cells of a person identifies infection in that individual. Besides being extremely sensitive, PCR tests can provide results in a few hours as opposed to days for culturing methods. They can also be used to detect infectious organisms that are difficult or impossible to grow in culture (e.g. tuberculosis, malaria) or are dangerous to handle (e.g. HIV/AIDS).

In the industrialized world, the use of PCR tests in the diagnosis of infectious diseases is increasing. Tests for HIV- 1, gonorrhea, pneumonia and herpes are already available. Recent advances are beginning to bring this powerful tool within reach of the developing world. For example, a group involved in the testing of infants for HIV-1 successfully processed and stored blood samples for up to several months on commercially available filter paper. A PCR test for three complexes of New World *Leishmania* (*Leishmania braziliensis*, *Leishmania mexicana*, and *Leishmania donovani*) – which cause a spectrum of diseases – was developed in Nicaragua and uses a technique known as multiplexing to test for more than one disease at once, saving both time and resources. Going a step beyond current practices in PCR are new *nanotechnology* methods for detecting infection at the molecular level, without the need for DNA amplification. One nanotechnique uses gold particles complexed with diagnostic DNA fragments that have the ability to bind to specific pathogen-associated DNA sequences. A sample of the patient's blood is placed between two tiny electrodes in the presence of the probe. When the probe and its target DNA sequence match, the gold particles close the circuit between the electrodes and produce a detectable signal. Not only is this approach more sensitive than conventional detection methods, it has the potential to be substantially more affordable.

While PCR tests are on their way to finding applications in developing countries, antibody-based applications are already highly suited to the developing world. *Antibodies* are molecules produced by the immune system in response to infection. They recognize and bind to proteins produced by pathogens. These proteins are known as antigens. Antibodies are specific, i.e. every antibody recognizes and binds to a specific type of antigen. This makes them an excellent tool for the diagnosis of infectious disease. In the last few years, the development of simple and rapid antibody-coated dipstick tests have increased the relevance of this technology for the developing world. Dipsticks can be used anywhere, without the need for laboratory facilities, running water or electricity. OptiMAL® is one of several antibody-based dipstick tests for malaria. During a malaria outbreak in Honduras, it rivalled the accuracy of microscopic analysis, the "gold standard" of malaria diagnosis. The Program for Appropriate Technology in Health, an international not for-profit organization committed to improving global health, has developed an HIV dipstick test that is now being produced by several private firms in developing countries. *Determine HIV-1/2* can diagnose both HIV-1 and HIV-2 based upon a reaction on a nitrocellulose strip between recombinant antigens and patient antibodies. The test is accurate and sensitive and has been successfully tested in the field in Ghana.

PATH is also developing dipsticks for the detection of malaria, TB and hepatitis C, among other diseases. Quidel has developed a dipstick test for *Streptococcus pneumoniae*, the most common cause of pneumonia. Monoclonal antibodies (mAb) are extremely specific antibodies. They are superior to antibodies harvested from human or animal serum because they are extraordinarily pure, show very high binding specificity and can be grown in large quantities. The drawback is that mammalian cell culture is expensive, so although the sensitivity and specificity of monoclonal antibodies are high, cost issues have prevented their widespread use in developing countries.

Plantibodies are monoclonal antibodies that are produced in genetically engineered plants and then extracted for medical use. They are a cheaper source of antibodies than those produced in mammalian cells. One estimate places the cost of a gram of plantibodies at less than 5% that of mammalian cell monoclonal antibodies. Another advantage is that they do not risk spreading animal diseases to humans. Plantibodies have been patented by Epicyte, a U.S. biotechnology company which plans to begin clinical trials of its anti-Herpes Simplex Virus 1 and 2 plantibody mixture, HX8. The company was recently awarded a grant from the US National Institutes of Health for the development of plantibodies against Human Papilloma Virus (HPV), which causes cervical cancer. Other companies have begun human trials of plantibodies for Hepatitis B, sexually transmitted diseases, and non-Hodgkin's lymphoma.

The Monoclonal Antibody

Culture Technique

The technique of monoclonal antibody culture involves three broad steps. The first step is to immunize a mouse with an antigen. When the mouse begins to produce antibodies to the antigen, its spleen is removed. Antibody-producing cells from the spleen are then fused with tumour cells (which grow and divide in vitro and are 'immortal'). Each hybrid cell produces identical antibody molecules. By allowing the hybrid cells to multiply in culture, it is possible to produce a population of cells, each of which produces identical antibody molecules. These antibodies are called "monoclonal antibodies" because they are produced by the identical offspring of a single antibody-producing cell. The new fused cell can also be re-injected into another mouse. This mouse produces pure monoclonal antibodies. The use of monoclonal antibodies for the diagnosis of infectious disease dates back to the early 1980s.

A New Test for Tuberculosis

New developments in diagnostic testing for tuberculosis indicate the diverse ways in which scientists are using the immune system for detecting the presence of pathogens in the blood. A major obstacle to controlling tuberculosis is the lack of a reliable diagnostic blood test. The treatment of TB relies upon the identification of tuberculosis infection by targeted tuberculin skin testing, the main drawback of which is low specificity. For example, the BCG vaccination and environmental mycobacterial exposure can both result in false-positive results.

In response to this shortcoming, researchers at Oxford University and the Wellcome Trust have developed a new test. This test targets cells in the blood that are produced by the immune system, called T-cells. The presence of specific T cells, detected by the rapid ex-vivo enzyme-linked immunospot (ELISPOT) assay for interferon-gamma, is a highly sensitive and specific indicator of infection in patients who have tuberculosis; its sensitivity is substantially higher than that for the skin test. This test is set to supersede the tuberculin skin test and improve the control and prevention of this resurgent disease. The test is simple, quick, and not confounded by TB vaccination. Doctors hope it will supersede the skin test in the next few years and transform the way TB is diagnosed and controlled.

As mentioned earlier, pathogen cells are associated with distinguishing molecules known as antigens, and antibodies can be used to detect the presence of antigens in a person's bloodstream. Similarly, antigens can also be used to detect antibodies. *Recombinant antigens* are genetically-engineered antigens mass-produced by fast-replicating organisms such as bacteria or yeast. (The term recombinant refers to the DNA produced when genetic information from more than one organism is 'recombined' in a laboratory process to form a hybrid molecule. A desired antigen is produced by incorporation of its DNA sequence into the DNA of a host bacterial cell). Like monoclonal antibodies, recombinant antigens also feature in simple handheld test devices capable of providing a diagnosis in a matter of minutes. These devices are particularly well suited to developing areas where clean water and electricity are not always accessible and people might have to travel significant distances to reach a medical facility.

Recombinant Vaccines

- Reduce child mortality
- Improve maternal health
- Combat HIV/AIDS, malaria and other diseases.

Recombinant vaccines can play an important part in achieving the fourth Millennium Development Goal, *Reduce child mortality* as well as to the fifth and sixth MDGs, *Improve maternal health* and *Combat HIV/AIDS, malaria and other diseases.* The hepatitis B vaccine saves the lives of millions of people, including children, every year, and many HIV vaccine candidates currently under investigation are recombinant vaccines.

Vaccines stimulate the body to produce a protective immune response and thereby reduce the likelihood of serious infection. They are arguably the most important medical advance of the last hundred years. Vaccination has resulted in the eradication of smallpox, the imminent eradication of polio, and a dramatic reduction in the prevalence of many other infectious diseases. Advances in vaccine research are expected to have an impact not only on communicable diseases, but also on non-communicable ones such as cancer.

Until a few decades ago, all vaccines consisted of either killed or inactivated ('attenuated') pathogens. Injection of this into a person would stimulate the person's immune system to produce antibodies against the foreign organism, thus conferring resistance to the pathogen in future infections. However, pathogen inactivation may sometimes be insufficient, so that vaccination with a live pathogen, even though it is weakened, carries a finite risk of causing a fatal infection. *Genetic engineering* (also known as *recombinant technology*) makes it possible to have single proteins of the pathogen produced in non-pathogenic microorganisms; injection of a person with these organisms stimulates antibody production against the foreign protein and therefore provides protection against the disease. The obvious advantage of this approach is the enhanced safety of the vaccine, since the single foreign protein cannot cause the disease. Recombinant vaccines made with only part of the genome of a pathogen are also known as subunit vaccines.

Recombinant vaccines may also prove to be cheaper than traditional vaccines because of innovative production methods and, in some cases, because improved storage characteristics may not require them to be refrigerated. Much progress is being made in recombinant vaccine development. A major roadblock is the long time it takes for clinical trials and regulatory approval. To date, the number of products on the market is quite limited. Researchers are currently working to develop techniques to overcome some of the other difficulties too, for example, correct presentation of recombinant antigens to the immune system and the limited lifetime of the engineered protein in the body.

Types of Recombinant Vaccines

Viral vector vaccines consist of a benign virus that has been genetically modified to contain genetic material belonging to the pathogen. After the vaccine has been injected, the virus attaches to the individual's cells and injects its genetic material into the cell's interior. The foreign genetic material gets incorporated into the cell's genome. The cell follows the genetic code and manufactures the antigens of interest, which trigger the immune system into producing a protective immune response.

Naked DNA vaccines, or plasmid DNA vaccines as they are also known, are very similar to viral vector vaccines. The key difference is that naked DNA vaccines use a different biological carrier, known as a plasmid, to introduce the antigen genes into the individual's cells. Plasmids are small circular molecules of DNA that are normally found in bacteria. They can easily enter cells and recruit the cell to translate their genetic information into protein. Advocates of this approach argue that developing naked DNA vaccines is potentially faster, cheaper and easier than other types of vaccines and, because DNA is heatstable, these vaccines are able to bypass the cold chain, a major cost barrier to efficient vaccine delivery.

Plant-derived vaccines are subunit vaccines synthesized by plants. Plants typically used are those that are easily engineered to express foreign proteins, such as the tomato or potato. After introducing the pathogen genes into the plant's DNA, the plant is given a signal to make the protein in its tissues. The antigens expressed by the plant are purified and can then be used as vaccines. In essence, the plants act as vaccine-factories. There are several advantages to plant-derived vaccines. They can be relatively inexpensive to produce, store, and transport and they could be grown locally, making them attractive for applications in developing countries. Researchers are making significant progress in the development of plant-derived vaccines. In comparison to the existing hepatitis B vaccine, a potato-derived vaccine was found to produce greater immunity in mice. Plant-derived vaccines are also being developed for several important causes of infant mortality, including infant diarrhea and measles.

Recombinant Vaccines in Development

Most HIV vaccines currently in clinical trials are recombinant vaccines. Currently there are 28 ongoing trials collectively involving 24 different vaccines. Of these, 8 are DNA-based, 8 use recombinant viral vectors, 5 are protein subunits and 3 are lipopeptides. An HIV viral vector vaccine based upon the gp120 antigen has shown encouraging results in a Phase II clinical trial with healthy volunteers. Just over half of all volunteers generated antibodies that neutralized HIV-1. When received in combination with an injection of gp120, the proportion rose to 94%. Phase III trials began in late 2003. In recent trials on Rhesus macaques, researchers assessed the protection conferred by recombinant forms of HIV gp120, a fusion protein constructed from HIV regulatory proteins Nef and Tat, and SIV Nef. Treatment with this recombinant multiantigen vaccine delayed the onset of AIDS in Rhesus monkeys for at least 2.5 years following infection with a simian-human hybrid virus (S-HIV).

The much-awaited initial results of a three-year multi-ethnic phase III trial of AIDSVAX by researchers at VaxGen Inc. have been disappointing. Produced in mammalian cell culture, AIDSVAX is a recombinant form of gp120. It is non-infectious and mimics proteins on the surface of two strains of HIV subtype B (prevalent in North America, Europe, Australia, Japan and Puerto Rico). The FDA would have considered approving the vaccine if it were 30% effective, but the reduction of infection among the entire sample of volunteers including all racial groups was only 3.8 %. The study did not show a statistically significant reduction of HIV infection within the study population as a whole, which was the primary endpoint of trial. Nonetheless, larger and statistically significant reductions were observed in some ethnic groups, especially among African-Americans, so further studies on this vaccine are warranted. A naked DNA vaccine against HIV/AIDS is currently being evaluated in The Gambia and England, with good results. The first multi-clad HIV vaccine to enter clinical trials is also a naked DNA vaccine. By preventing infection by the three most important subtypes of the virus around the world, it is hoped that this vaccine would be effective in both developing and developed countries.

All said and done, however, the progress of HIV vaccine development has been slow and disappointing. After 10 years of work in this area, scientists now believe that live, attenuated vaccines may be more appropriate for the fastevolving and diverse HIV.

The story of recombinant vaccines against malaria is more promising. A subunit vaccine known as RTS,S/AS02 was recently shown to provide protection against natural malaria infection in adults in a clinical trial in the Gambia, with 71% of the participants protected from infection for the first 9 weeks of the study. Clinical trials on children in both The Gambia and Mozambique are now underway. Another subunit vaccine protected four of five monkeys from a lethal injection of malaria. This particular vaccine is synthesized by mice and excreted in their milk. The developers have expressed interest in creating transgenic goats for large-scale production. Tuberculosis claims at least 2 million lives every year. Researchers are actively working towards a potent TB vaccine. 72 Progress to date includes a subunit vaccine based upon the Mtb8.4 surface antigen that protected mice from virulent TB infection.

Hepatitis B affects approximately one third of the world's population and is associated with liver cancer. Tomatoes and lettuce have been genetically engineered to produce hepatitis B surface antigens, and these appear to induce an immune reaction similar to hepatitis B proteins isolated from infected humans. Scientists are developing plant-derived vaccines against the major causes of infant diarrhea. For instance, researchers successfully produced a strain of corn that expresses an antigen associated with enterotoxic *E. coli*. Mice that were fed the corn exhibited elevated levels of antibodies in their blood, and showed resistance to infection. Also, the gene for the highly antigenic, but non-toxic, beta chain of the cholera toxin has been expressed in alfalfa, and mice fed with this alfalfa showed an immune response against cholera toxin. However, it will probably take many years of careful experimentation before such vaccines are approved for human use.

Bioremediation

- Combat HIV/AIDS, malaria and other diseases
- Ensure environmental sustainability.

Technologies for environmental improvement (sanitation, clean water, bioremediation) were ranked fourth in the list of technologies to improve health in developing countries.

Bioremediation has direct significance to the seventh MDG, *Ensure environmental sustainability* but it also has impact on the health-related goals.

Bioremediation is the use of bacteria or plants to clean up the environment. Reduction of pollution in water supplies and in the food chain will help to reduce mortality and improve health. There are two main types of pollution threatening the health and well-being of human populations: organic waste and heavy metals such as lead, mercury and cadmium. Bacteria can detoxify both. Plants can break down most forms of organic waste, but, with very feexceptions, are usually unable to metabolize heavy metals.

On the other hand they can store harmful metals in their tissues and therefore make it easier to collect, harvest and even recycle metal waste.

Water contaminated by human waste harbors large amounts of pathogenic organisms and has been implicated in the transmission of cholera, typhoid, hepatitis A another waterborne diseases. Sewage treatment can dramatically reduce the incidence of these diseases. Bioremediation techniques can augment conventional chemical sewage treatment. A number of low-cost alternatives to conventional sewage treatment have been developed. One such system is now in use in

Southern China. It uses floating rafts called Restorers to supply beneficial microorganisms to a canal contaminated with human waste. In fact, this floating ecological treatment engine has now been transformed into a garden featuring over 10 species of native Chinese wetland plants.

Bioremediation can also be used to reduce environmental pollution associated with heavy industries, including oil spills, acid mine drainage, and radioactive waste. In 1989 the tanker Exxon Valdez released 11 million gallons of oil off the coast of Alaska, affecting approximately 2000 km of shoreline.

Through the addition of extra nutrients to the beach, crews were able to enhance local bacterial and algal populations and take advantage of their ability to degrade petroleum.

Acid mine drainage is associated with the leakage of contaminated water from mining sites. The drainage is toxic for both humans and the surrounding environment.

Constructed wetlands are a common low-cost, sustainable solution to this problem. The area is artificially saturated with water, plant species are introduced, and these eventually lower the acidity and the metal concentrations at the site.

The bacterium *Deinococcus radiodurans* has the ability to thrive in environments with 300 times the fatal dose of radiation for humans. Researchers have genetically engineered

D. radiodurans to express several genes associated with mercury detoxification. The recombinant bacterium has been shown to metabolize mercury while being bombarded by high levels of radiation, suggesting that bioremediation may be able to aid in the process of radioactive waste cleanup.

Bioremediation can also help to clean up mosquito-infested water and control the spread of malaria. For example, the malaria-carrying *Anopheles* mosquito has developed resistance to chemical insecticides. Many anti-malarial prophylactics that were once effective are now less reliable, not to mention expensive for many people in developing countries.

Peru has one of the highest rates of malaria in all of Latin America. Canada's International Development Research Centre (IDRC) has supported research at the Instituto de Medicina Tropical "Alexander Von Humboldt" in Lima to explore the use of coconuts in the fight against malaria. Researchers at the Institute have developed an ingenious method to biologically control mosquitoes that is simple, inexpensive, and an environmentally safe alternative to insecticides. It involves the use of coconuts used to culture bacteria that are toxic to mosquito larvae but harmless to people and other organisms. *Bacillus thuringiensis* var. *israelensis* H-14 (*Bti*) is a spore-forming bacterium that produces a toxin lethal to mosquito larvae. Imported *Bti* cultures are expensive, but as this project shows *Bti* can be cultured locally and cheaply using coconuts, which are both cheap and plentiful in many tropical areas. *Bti* is introduced via cotton swabs into the coconut and allowed to incubate inside the coconut for a few days. The nut is then broken and tossed into ponds where mosquitoes breed. The mosquito larvae eat the bacteria and are killed. A typical pond needs only two or three coconuts for each treatment – usually lasting 2 months.

Sequencing Pathogen Genomes

- Combat HIV/AIDS, malaria and other diseases.

The sequencing of pathogen genomes has direct relevance to the fourth Millennium Development Goal, *Combat HIV/AIDS, malaria and other diseases.* The task force for this MDG has prepared documents on HIV/AIDS, malaria and TB that take an in-depth look at the science, public health needs and medical interventions, and the social and economic issues and consequences of these devastating diseases. Pathogen genomics can also contribute to the search for a solution of these diseases.

Sequencing a genome involves discovering and recording the entire sequence of nucleotides in an organism's DNA. DNA codes for proteins, which are the mainstay of structure and biochemical function in all organisms. Knowing the sequence of a pathogen's genome is therefore helpful in unraveling its biology and discovering effective ways of controlling its relationship with humans.

Most sequencing strategies are based upon a technique known as the dideoxy or Sanger method. Small-scale sequencing projects can be done manually, but large-scale projects (such as the sequencing of an entire genome) require high-throughput automated DNA sequencing machines. Major sequencing projects use many automated sequencing machines simultaneously, yielding millions of bases of sequence data per day. These data must be stored, managed and analysed by computers and this requirement has given rise to an entirely new field in biology -bioinformatics.

Knowing the sequence of a pathogen's genome can rapidly accelerate the process of drug discovery. Comparative genomics is a method that compares the genomes of different organisms in order to apply information known about one organism to another. For example, in a comparison of disease-causing and benign strains of the same organism, genes unique to the pathogenic strain are likely to play an important role in pathogenesis, and the proteins for which they code may make excellent drug targets. Alternatively, if one pathogen has a gene that is a known drug target, a comparative genomics search might reveal a similar gene, and therefore a potential drug target, in another pathogen.

A serious health concern worldwide is the emergence of pathogen resistance to previously effective drugs. Analysis of pathogen genomes could reveal the genes that play a role in helping these organisms develop drug resistance and point researchers in the direction of treatments that can overcome the action of these genes. For example, scientists can compare the genomes of resistant and nonresistant strains, or analyze the genes at work in the drug resistant stage of an organism's lifecycle.

In addition to spurring novel drug discovery, pathogen genomics has also given a boost to the development of vaccines. Researchers can search the genome of infectious organisms for gene sequences characteristic of antigens. For example, scientists have discovered vaccine candidates for a particularly virulent strain of meningitis, a potentially fatal bacterial infection. Of the 570 antigens found, 85 showed promise when used to immunize mice.

Female-controlled Protection Against Sexually Transmitted Infections (STIS)

- Promote gender equality and empower women
- Improve maternal health
- Reduce child mortality.

Genomics and other biotechnologies are enabling the development of a number of new forms of female-controlled protection against STIs, such as recombinant vaccines, monoclonal antibodies and new approaches to the development of vaginal microbicides. These technologies can help to meet the sixth MDG *Combat HIV/AIDS, malaria and other diseases* and even the third MDG, *Promote gender equality and empower women* with an indirect effect on other health MDGs: e.g. *Reducing child mortality* by *Improving maternal health*.

The global burden of STIs is felt most heavily by women. A decade ago, the World Bank ranked STIs as the second major cause of ill health among women aged 15 to 44, accounting for 8.9% of their disease burden, compared to 1.5% in men. For various reasons – socio-economic, cultural and biological – women are more vulnerable to infection than men. Women with STIs often bear heavy social stigma, and they often have neither the time nor the money to seek health care. Rising infection in women also increases the incidence of transmission from mother to newborn. Despite the seriousness of this problem, women possess few means of protection. The condom requires male consent, which many women living in patriarchal societies find hard to negotiate in their relationships. Although the female condom has been greeted with enthusiasm by women in poor countries, its cost and indiscreetness make it a less than ideal option. Vaginal microbicides are one attractive alternative. They are gel or cream formulations of chemical compounds that block the transmission of infection across the vaginal wall. Researchers are actively involved in developing safe and effective vaginal microbicides.

More recently, researchers in India have developed a potato rich in all essential amino acids. This potato contains the gene AmA1 that codes for the protein albumin, which contains high levels of all amino acids that the body is incapable of making on its own (i.e. essential amino-acids). It gives ordinary potatoes a third more protein than normal, including substantial amounts of the essential amino acids lysine and methionine. Deficiency in these can have an adverse effect on development in children. This enriched potato is also particularly relevant for India, where a large percentage of the population is vegetarian. The AmA1 gene was obtained from the amaranth plant which grows in South America. The potato is in the final stages of testing, and it has been submitted for official approval. Scientists say that the protein-rich genetically modified "protato" could help combat malnutrition among the country's poorest children. Researchers have also inserted into lettuce the gene for the enzyme GLOase, which converts a precursor molecule into Vitamin C. They observed up to a seven-fold increase for Vitamin C in the plant's tissues. Vitamin C is a powerful antioxidant and is associated with reduced risks of cancer, cardiovascular disease and other diseases.

Genetic modification and traditional breeding both change the characteristics of an organism, but in different ways. In traditional breeding, the introduction of a gene into an organism by cross breeding different strains of the same species is a trial-and-error process that takes a long time. Genetic modification makes it possible to introduce new genes more rapidly and more precisely than traditional breeding and enables the introduction of new genes from different species. In many cases, traditional breeding alone is able to improve the nutritional value of a crop. In fact farmers have used traditional breeding over thousands of years to convert the wild, almost inedible forms of rice and wheat into the familiar foods we eat today. However, genetic modification has the advantage of speed and relative control. This approach has its advantages and disadvantages. An obvious disadvantage is that the introduced foreign genes may cause unknown gene-gene or gene-environment interactions. Ecological concerns include risks to human and animal health, food safety, and unforeseen consequences of the spreading of foreign genes into the natural environment. Gene-flow, the natural spread of genetic traits when a plant variety is introduced into the environment, is in itself not alarming, but the potential introduction of cross-species genes and the spread of these genes that confer novel traits upon related weeds or crops could be.

However, it is important to note that all plant breeding, whether traditional or through genetic engineering, can produce unexpected results. Some scientists recommend that extensive testing and careful monitoring are necessary for the world to reap the benefits of this technology while avoiding any potential risks. Others argue that all plant varieties, whether GM or not, should be subject to the same stringent standards. a, b Although GM enriched crops are considered by many to be extremely important for health in developing countries, there are some concerns regarding their use. There is, for example, evidence that Golden Rice may not be a very good source of Vitamin A. Specifically, people with diarrheal diseases, which are common in the developing world, are unable to efficiently absorb Vitamin A from the rice. Critics also maintain that GM enriched crops are not the answer to the problems of hunger and malnutrition, which are the outcomes of distributional problems. Several organizations are actively researching these issues. The Food and Agriculture Organization of the United Nations and the World Health Organization jointly recommend the thorough evaluation of GM foods for safety and nutritional value before consumption or releasing the foods into the environment.

Genomics Capacity Building

The genomics revolution will have an impact not only on health care, but also on agriculture (genetically modified organisms) and economics (pharmaceutical industry). Social implications will also be broad, as illustrated by Pedro Leon's description of the genetic basis of deafness as well as recent Costa Rican legislation on compulsory DNA testing so that children have the "right to know their fathers." Despite the publicity and hype, genomics is not a panacea or magic bullet. Whatever happens, biotechnology will not solve deep-seated problems like poverty for those living under $1-2 per day, who need drinking water, food, and livelihoods. Genomics is inherently controversial because it is central to sex, money, reproduction, race, and privacy. Warnings were issued about eugenics, cloning, discrimination, and genetic determinism. Even without genomics, we are witnessing some technological abuse, like pre-natal sex selection in some Asian societies. Public worries about "Frankenfoods" may indeed become real worries about "biological Frankensteins." These issues set the stage for three central Conference challenges, in my opinion. What is really bothering us about the genomics revolution? What should we do? And how can WHO play its pre-eminent role in genomics and world health?

What's the Problem?

The genomics revolution has provoked genuine disquiet, sometimes passion and even fear. Discomfort could come from insecurity about the loss of control over our lives in uncertain times. History is not entirely reassuring in this regard. Throughout human history, warfare and profits have powerfully propelled technology development. Indeed, I was surprised that the anthrax bioterrorism attack in the United States did not receive more attention. We know that powerful technologies with destructive potential, like nuclear power, can unleash unintentional consequences of far greater import than planned change. Once the genie is out of the bottle, it's hard to put it back in. Bruce Lewenstein presented survey data of public perceptions about genomics, mostly from rich countries. Public awareness is growing, but "genetic illiteracy" and popular hype are also prevalent. As I listened, I began to interpret a new meaning to "know thyself." That used to signal reflections about my personality, my psychology, and my behaviour. With the genomics revolution, know thyself now prompts reflections about my genes and biology! A recurring theme underlying our worries is social inequity. Inequity differs from inequality in that the latter describes objective disparity while the former introduces a normative lens on whether such inequality is perceived as fair or unfair. Inequity, therefore, is a moral judgment about the nature of inequality in society. Concern about inequity is escalating, in part, because of the globalization of private markets. Rapid transnational flows of money, goods, services, technology, culture, and people are introducing new vulnerabilities, uncertain risks, and heightened public consciousness about distant people in a shrinking world. With the exception of malaria, a greatly neglected disease, the three other infections discussed in our breakout sessions may be characterized as "diseases of globalization," because their emergence or re-emergence is associated with rapid transnational flows. The global spread of HIV/AIDS was certainly associated with global movement. Tuberculosis, also a major neglected disease, has increased dramatically due to HIV-compromised host immunity. Resurgence of dengue fever is due, in part, to movements of people and goods that facilitate the transmission of the vector-borne virus.

Jose Maria Cantu predicted that the "fight of the 21st century" will be between the "WHO and WHM" (world health market). He suggested a fundamental tension between WHO's mission of equitable world health and inequitable forces generated by competitive private markets. Because the poor lack purchasing power, market-driven health services will not address their health care needs. Lack of a profitable market provides little incentives for industry to pursue R&D to develop technologies against diseases of the poor. Peter Singer and Abdullah Daar urged that actions be taken to preempt a looming "genomic divide." Some have described this phenomenon as a "market failure," implying that markets serve well most purposes but leave a few social gaps. I would prefer calling the problem a "social failure," since even if markets were to function perfectly, they would not address the fundamental deficiency of the inability of the poor to command goods and services through the marketplace.

What Should We Do?

How do we produce essential global public goods? How do we shape markets to generate more equitable outcomes? I address these two questions and also reflect on lessons from Cuba today and China yesterday.

Certain goods wanted and needed by everyone, like clean air and public parks, cannot be produced by private markets. Genomics R&D for technologies against neglected infectious diseases fit into this category. The term "public goods" describes these non-rival and non-excludable goods. How then can we produce global public goods? Given their non-market nature, public goods are appropriately generated by public action and public financing.

R&D, however, is expensive and time-consuming, requiring a strong infrastructure of skilled people, facilities, equipment and supplies. David Webber reported that members of the International Federation of Pharmaceutical Manufacturers Association invest $40 billion annually in R&D. Global imbalances of investments underscore the obstacles faced by many developing countries. According to Tikki Pang, of an estimated $5 billion invested annually in genomics research, $3 billion is private and 75% is in the United States, which also registers about 80% of genomics patents worldwide. Some developing countries – Cuba, Thailand, India, and China – are emerging contributors to genomics research. But, what about other developing countries? Michael Wilson described a "catch-22" situation in Ghana of a vicious cycle of weak financing, little research, few facilities, no jobs, and ultimately out-migration of skilled scientists. To remedy the R&D gap, two dozen so-called public-private partnerships (PPPs) have been created. These PPPs mostly aim to produce public goods in health. Many believe that these "push" mechanisms (production of neglected vaccine and drugs) must be balanced by "pull" forces (like subsidized vaccine purchase funds) to correct for market failure.

Can markets be shaped to generate fairer outcomes? Severe inequity is not a preordained outcome of markets that involve millions of individual and collective decisions. Markets, however, are social institutions governed by humanly constructed ground rules. Depending upon ground rules, it is possible to generate various levels of fairness. Weak initial capability upon entering competitive markets is one example of handicaps faced by many developing countries. Many also feel aggrieved because these disadvantages are historically inherited, and developing countries often lack the political and economic clout to negotiate better entry conditions.

Another ground rule is intellectual property rights (IPR). Lalji Singh described the cultural alarm of Indians as foreigners patented indigenous plants —the neem tree, turmeric spices, and Basmati rice. The controversy over IPR will not simply go away. George Soros in his recent book, "Globalization," describes how IPR in today's knowledge-based economy should be treated differently than earlier technology eras. In the industrial revolution, either new or some commonly-owned assets became privatized – for example, telegraph lines, railway tracks, subsurface petroleum, and manufacturing machines. Intellectual property in a knowledge-based economy poses different challenges to balance incentives for innovation, appropriate returns to an inventor, and economic progress. These historical dimensions of IPR should not distract us from practical intermediate steps that can be taken to reduce inequities in IPR management.

Bibek Debroy argued that wholesale changes are neither likely nor necessary, nor must solutions be conflictual. One example of positive adjustment is ensuring royalty returns to affected genetic lineages for research participation in Costa Rica. Another potentially very significant advance is Management of Intellectual Property in Health R&D (MIHR), recently established by the Rockefeller Foundation to assist non-profit organizations negotiate IPR, licensing, and other arrangements.

As described by Luis Herrera and his colleagues, Cuba is an admirable health success story. Its 11 million people enjoy an average life expectancy of 76 years and an infant mortality rate of 6 per 1,000 livebirths — roughly equivalent to Canada and superior to the United States. As a basic human right, health care is universal, accessible, and free.

Cuba also has adopted an "internationalist public health" policy that exported 2,600 health workers to other countries. With universal literacy, 58 universities and 115 research institutes, Cuba has one physician per 179 population and more than one teacher per 50 people. Its rich human resources are important to a state-led biotechnology sector, which has received strong political commitment and sustained investments. The state-led sector pursues vertical integration of pharmaceutical research-product-marketing, called by Dr. Herrera, a "closed cycle strategy." Drs. Moreno and Mauri described how Cuba also pursues IPR protection and marketing through "strategic alliances" with foreign firms. In the United States, we have a market-led biotechnology sector. Of course, the public sector through the NIH provides nearly $20 billion of funding for basic research that is tapped by the private sector. Other countries, for example Thailand, have their own unique mix of state-led and market-led R&D. The lesson here is that different national patterns of R&D systems are possible, even as all nations compete in a global economy.

Chapter 3

Genetic Code

The genetic code is the set of rules by which information encoded in genetic material (DNA or mRNA sequences) is translated into proteins (amino acid sequences) by living cells. The code defines a mapping between tri-nucleotide sequences, called codons, and amino acids. With some exceptions, a triplet codon in a nucleic acid sequence specifies a single amino acid. Because the vast majority of genes are encoded with exactly the same code, this particular code is often referred to as the canonical or standard genetic code, or simply *the* genetic code, though in fact there are many variant codes. For example, protein synthesis in human mitochondria relies on a genetic code that differs from the standard genetic code.

Not all genetic information is stored using the genetic code. All organisms' DNA contains regulatory sequences, intergenic segments, and chromosomal structural areas that can contribute greatly to phenotype. Those elements operate under sets of rules that are distinct from the codon-to-amino acid paradigm underlying the genetic code.

Discovery

After the structure of DNA was deciphered by James Watson, Francis Crick, Maurice Wilkins and Rosalind Franklin, serious efforts to understand the nature of the encoding of proteins began. George Gamow postulated that a three-letter code must be employed to encode the 20 standard amino acids used by living cells to encode proteins, because 3 is the smallest integer n such that 4 is at least 20.

The fact that codons consist of three DNA bases was first demonstrated in the Crick, Brenner et al. experiment. The first elucidation of a codon was done by Marshall Nirenberg and Heinrich J. Matthaei in 1961 at the National Institutes of Health. They used a cell-free system to translate a poly-uracil RNA sequence (i.e., UUUUU...) and discovered that the polypeptide that they had synthesized consisted of only the amino acid phenylalanine. They thereby deduced that the codon UUU specified the amino acid phenylalanine. This was followed by experiments in the laboratory of Severo Ochoa demonstrating that the poly-adenine RNA sequence (AAAAA...) coded for the polypeptide, poly-lysine. and the poly-cytosine RNA sequence (CCCCC...) coded for the polypeptide, poly-proline. Therefore the codon AAA specified the amino acid lysine, and the codon CCC specified the amino acid proline. Using different copolymers most of the remaining codons were then determined. Extending this work, Nirenberg and Philip Leder revealed the triplet nature of the genetic code and allowed the codons of the standard genetic code to be deciphered. In these experiments various combinations of mRNA were passed through a filter which contained ribosomes, the components of cells that translate RNA into protein. Unique triplets promoted the binding of specific tRNAs to the ribosome. Leder and Nirenberg were able to determine the sequences of 54 out of 64 codons in their experiments.

Subsequent work by Har Gobind Khorana identified the rest of the genetic code. Shortly thereafter, Robert W. Holley determined the structure of transfer RNA (tRNA), the adapter molecule that facilitates the process of translating RNA into protein. This work was based upon earlier studies by Severo Ochoa, who received the Nobel prize in 1959 for his work on the enzymology of RNA synthesis. In 1968, Khorana, Holley and Nirenberg received the Nobel Prize in Physiology or Medicine for their work.

Transfer of Information Via the Genetic Code

The genome of an organism is inscribed in DNA, or in the case of some viruses, RNA. The portion of the genome that codes for a protein or an RNA is referred to as a gene. Those genes that code for proteins are composed of tri-nucleotide units called codons, each coding for a single amino acid. Each nucleotide sub-unit consists of a phosphate, deoxyribose sugar and one of the 4 nitrogenous nucleobases. The purine bases adenine (A) and guanine (G) are larger and consist of two aromatic rings. The pyrimidine bases cytosine (C) and thymine (T) are smaller and consist of only one aromatic ring. In the double-helix configuration, two strands of DNA are joined to each other by hydrogen bonds in an arrangement known as base pairing. These bonds almost always form between an adenine base on one strand and a thymine on the other strand and between a cytosine base on one strand and a guanine base on the other. This means that the number of A and T residues will be the same in a given double helix, as will the number of G and C residues. In RNA, thymine (T) is replaced by uracil (U), and the deoxyribose is substituted by ribose.

Each protein-coding gene is transcribed into a template molecule of the related polymer RNA, known as messenger RNA or mRNA. This, in turn, is translated on the ribosome into an amino acid chain or polypeptide. The process of translation requires transfer RNAs specific for individual amino acids with the amino acids covalently attached to them, guanosine triphosphate as an energy source, and a number of translation factors. tRNAs have anticodons complementary to the codons in mRNA and can be "charged" covalently with amino acids at their 3' terminal CCA ends. Individual tRNAs are charged with specific amino acids by enzymes known as aminoacyl tRNA synthetases, which have high specificity for both their cognate amino acids and tRNAs. The high specificity of these enzymes is a major reason why the fidelity of protein translation is maintained.

There are $4^3 = 64$ different codon combinations possible with a triplet codon of three nucleotides; all 64 codons are assigned for either amino acids or stop signals during translation. If, for example, an RNA sequence, UUUAAACCC is considered and the reading frame starts with the first U (by convention, 5' to 3'), there are three codons, namely, UUU, AAA and CCC, each of which specifies one amino acid. This RNA sequence will be translated into an amino acid sequence, three amino acids long. A comparison may be made with computer science, where the codon is similar to a word, which is the standard "chunk" for handling data (like one amino acid of a protein), and a nucleotide is similar to a bit, in that it is the smallest unit.

Salient Features

Sequence Reading Frame

A codon is defined by the initial nucleotide from which translation starts. For example, the string GGGAAACCC, if read from the first position, contains the codons GGG, AAA and CCC; and, if read from the second position, it contains the codons GGA and AAC; if read starting from the third position, GAA and ACC. Every sequence can thus be read in three reading frames, each of which will produce a different amino acid sequence (in the given example, Gly-Lys-Pro, Gly-Asn, or Glu-Thr, respectively). With double-stranded DNA there are six possible reading frames, three in the forward orientation on one strand and three reverse on the opposite strand. The actual frame in which a protein sequence is translated is defined by a start codon, usually the first AUG codon in the mRNA sequence.

Start/Stop Codons

Translation starts with a chain initiation codon (start codon). Unlike stop codons, the codon alone is not sufficient to begin the process. Nearby sequences (such as the Shine-Dalgarno sequence in *E. coli*) and initiation factors are also required to start translation. The most common start codon is AUG which is read as methionine or, in bacteria, as formylmethionine. Alternative start codons (depending on the organism), include "GUG" or "UUG", which normally code for valine or leucine, respectively. However, when used as a start codon, these alternative start codons are translated as methionine or formylmethionine.

The three stop codons have been given names: UAG is *amber*, UGA is *opal* (sometimes also called *umber*), and UAA is *ochre*. "Amber" was named by discoverers Richard Epstein and Charles Steinberg after their friend Harris Bernstein, whose last name means "amber" in German. The other two stop codons were named "ochre" and "opal" in order to keep the "color names" theme. Stop codons are also called "termination" or "nonsense" codons and they signal release of the nascent polypeptide from the ribosome due to binding of release factors in the absence of cognate tRNAs with anticodons complementary to these stop signals.

Effect of Mutations

During the process of DNA replication, errors occasionally occur in the polymerization of the second strand. These errors, called mutations, can have an impact on the phenotype of an organism, especially if they occur within the protein coding sequence of a gene. Error rates are usually very low—1 error in every 10–100 million bases—due to the "proofreading" ability of DNA polymerases.

Missense mutations and nonsense mutations are examples of point mutations, which can cause genetic diseases such as sickle-cell disease and thalassemia respectively. Clinically important missense mutations generally change the properties of the coded amino acid residue between being basic, acidic polar or non-polar, whereas nonsense mutations result in a stop codon.

Mutations that disrupt the reading frame sequence by indels (insertions or deletions) of a non-multiple of 3 nucleotide bases are known as frameshift mutations. These mutations usually result in a completely different translation from the original, and are also very likely to cause a stop codon to be read, which truncates the creation of the protein. These mutations may impair the function of the resulting protein, and are thus rare in *in vivo* protein-coding sequences. One reason inheritance of frameshift mutations is rare is that if the protein being translated is essential for growth under the selective pressures the organism faces, absence of a functional protein may cause death before the organism is viable. Frameshift mutations may result in severe genetic diseases such as Tay-Sachs disease.

Although most mutations that change protein sequences are harmful or neutral, some mutations have a positive effect on an organism. These mutations may enable the mutant organism to withstand particular environmental stresses better than wild-type organisms, or reproduce more quickly. In these cases a mutation will tend to become more common in a population through natural selection. Viruses that use RNA as their genetic material have rapid mutation rates, which can be an advantage since these viruses will evolve constantly and rapidly, and thus evade the defensive responses of e.g. the human immune system. In large populations of asexually reproducing organisms, for example, E. coli, multiple beneficial mutations may co-occur, causing competition among them, this phenomenon is called clonal interference.

Degeneracy of the Genetic Code

The genetic code has redundancy but no ambiguity. For example, although codons GAA and GAG both specify glutamic acid (redundancy), neither of them specifies any other amino acid (no ambiguity). The codons encoding one amino acid may differ in any of their three positions. For example the amino acid glutamic acid is specified by GAA and GAG codons (difference in the third position), the amino acid leucine is specified by UUA, UUG, CUU, CUC, CUA, CUG codons (difference in the first or third position), while the amino acid serine is specified by UCA, UCG, UCC, UCU, AGU, AGC (difference in the first, second or third position).

A position of a codon is said to be a fourfold degenerate site if any nucleotide at this position specifies the same amino acid. For example, the third position of the glycine codons (GGA, GGG, GGC, GGU) is a fourfold degenerate site, because all nucleotide substitutions at this site are synonymous; i.e., they do not change the amino acid. Only the third positions of some codons may be fourfold degenerate. A position of a codon is said to be a twofold degenerate site if only two of four possible nucleotides at this position specify the same amino acid. For example, the third position of the glutamic acid codons (GAA, GAG) is a twofold degenerate site. In twofold degenerate sites, the equivalent nucleotides are always either two purines (A/G) or two pyrimidines (C/U), so only transversional substitutions (purine to pyrimidine or pyrimidine to purine) in twofold degenerate sites are nonsynonymous. A position of a codon is said to be a non-degenerate site if any mutation at this position results in amino acid substitution. There is only one threefold degenerate site where changing to three of the four nucleotides may have no effect on the amino acid (depending on what it is changed to), while changing to the fourth possible nucleotide always results in an amino acid substitution. This is the third position of an isoleucine codon: AUU, AUC, or AUA all encode isoleucine, but AUG encodes methionine. In computation this position is often treated as a twofold degenerate site.

There are three amino acids encoded by six different codons: serine, leucine, and arginine. Only two amino acids are specified by a single codon. One of these is the amino-acid methionine, specified by the codon AUG, which also specifies the start of translation; the other is tryptophan, specified by the codon UGG. The degeneracy of the genetic code is what accounts for the existence of synonymous mutations.

Degeneracy results because a triplet code designates 20 amino acids and a stop codon. Because there are four bases, triplet codons are required to produce at least 21 different codes. For example, if there were two bases per codon, then only 16 amino acids could be coded for ($4^2=16$). Because at least 21 codes are required, then 4^3 gives 64 possible codons, meaning that some degeneracy must exist.

These properties of the genetic code make it more fault-tolerant for point mutations. For example, in theory, fourfold degenerate codons can tolerate any point mutation at the third position, although codon usage bias restricts this in practice in many organisms; twofold degenerate codons can tolerate one out of the three possible point mutations at the third position. Since transition mutations (purine to purine or pyrimidine to pyrimidine mutations) are more likely than transversion (purine to pyrimidine or vice-versa) mutations, the equivalence of purines or that of pyrimidines at twofold degenerate sites adds a further fault-tolerance.

A practical consequence of redundancy is that some errors in the genetic code only cause a silent mutation or an error that would not affect the protein because the hydrophilicity or hydrophobicity is maintained by equivalent substitution of amino acids; for example, a codon of NUN (where N = any nucleotide) tends to code for hydrophobic amino acids. NCN yields amino acid residues that are small in size and moderate in hydropathy; NAN encodes average size hydrophilic residues. These tendencies may result from the shared ancestry of the aminoacyl tRNA synthetases related to these codons.

Even so, single point mutations can still cause dysfunctional proteins. For example, a mutated hemoglobin gene causes sickle-cell disease. In the mutant hemoglobin a hydrophilic glutamate (Glu) is substituted by the hydrophobic valine (Val), that is, GAA or GAG becomes GUA or GUG. The substitution of glutamate by valine reduces the solubility of â-globin which causes hemoglobin to form linear polymers linked by the hydrophobic interaction between the valine groups causing sickle-cell deformation of erythrocytes. Sickle-cell disease is generally not caused by a *de novo* mutation. Rather it is selected for in malarial regions (in a way similar to thalassemia), as heterozygous people have some resistance to the malarial *Plasmodium* parasite (heterozygote advantage).

These variable codes for amino acids are allowed because of modified bases in the first base of the anticodon of the tRNA, and the base-pair formed is called a wobble base pair. The modified bases include inosine and the Non-Watson-Crick U-G basepair.

Variations to the Standard Genetic Code

While slight variations on the standard code had been predicted earlier, none were discovered until 1979, when researchers studying human mitochondrial genes discovered they used an alternative code. Many slight variants have been discovered since, including various alternative mitochondrial codes, as well as small variants such as *Mycoplasma* translating the codon UGA as tryptophan and *Candida* species translating CUG as a serine rather than a leucine. In bacteria and archaea, GUG and UUG are common start codons. However, in rare cases, certain specific proteins may use alternative initiation (start) codons not normally used by that species.

In certain proteins, non-standard amino acids are substituted for standard stop codons, depending upon associated signal sequences in the messenger RNA: UGA can code for selenocysteine and UAG can code for pyrrolysine as discussed in the relevant articles. Selenocysteine is now viewed as the 21st amino acid, and pyrrolysine is viewed as the 22nd.

Notwithstanding these differences, all known codes have strong similarities to each other, and the coding mechanism is the same for all organisms: three-base codons, tRNA, ribosomes, reading the code in the same direction and translating the code three letters at a time into sequences of amino acids.

Expanded Genetic Code

An expanded genetic code refers to an artificially modified genetic code in which one or more specific codons have been allocated to encode an amino acid which is not among the twenty/twentytwo found in nature.

In order to understand how expansion of the genetic code is achieved, the translational mechanism catalysed by ribosomes should be considered: the central parts are the transfer RNAs (tRNA) which are used as keys to decode a three nucleotide code on the RNA being translated into its equivalent amino acid. To do this the tRNA recognises a specific codon thanks to a complementary sequence called the anticodon on one of its loops.

As a result generally there are one (or more) tRNAs for each codon (or group of degenerate codons). The encoding of a codon to its amino acid is a result of the aminoacyl tRNA synthetase which adds the aminoacyl group to its allocated tRNA.

However, the aminoacyl tRNA synthetase often recognises a specific motif irrespective of the anticodon, meaning that if the anticodon were to be mutated the encoding of that amino acid would change to a new codon.

For successful translation of a novel amino acid, the codon to which the amino acid is reassigned must be free or unfavoured and the novel tRNA and synthetase set (called the orthogonal set when including the codon) must not crosstalk with the endogenous tRNA and synthetase sets, while still being functionally compatible with the ribosome and other components of the translation apparatus. The tRNA synthetase pair is taken from a distant organism, generally from a different domain, and the active site of the synthetase is modified to accept the non-natural amino acid.

The possibility of reassigning codons was realized by Normanly et al. in 1990 when a viable mutant strain of E. coli read through the amber codon. As a result the amber codon became the choice codon to be assigned a novel amino acid. Later, in the Schultz lab the tRNATyr/tyrosyl-tRNA synthetase (TyrRS) from Methanococcus jannaschii was used to introduce a tyrosine instead of STOP, the default value of the amber codon. As mentioned, this was possible because of the differences between the endogenous bacterial synthases and the orthologous archeal synthase which do not recognise each other.

Directed Evolution

Several methods for selecting the synthetase which accepts only the non natural amino acid have been developed. One of which is by using a combination of positive and negative selection

Some amino acids which have been added in order to label protein.

This orthologous set can then be mutated and screened through directed evolution to accept a different, even novel, amino acid. Mutations to the plasmid containing the pair can be introduced by error-prone PCR or through degenerate primers for the synthetase's active site.

Selection involves multiple rounds of a two-step process, where the plasmid is transferred into cells expressing chloramphenicol acetyl transferase with a premature amber codon.

In the presence of toxic chloramphenicol and the non-natural amino acid, the surviving cells will have overridden the amber codon using the orthogonal tRNA aminoacylated with either the standard amino acids or the non-natural one. To remove the former, the plasmid is inserted into cells with a barnase gene (toxic) with a premature amber codon but without the non-natural amino acid, removing all the orthogonal synthases which do not specifically recognize the non-natural amino acid.

In addition to the recoding of the tRNA to a different codon, they can be mutated to recognize a four base codon, allowing additional free coding options. The non natural amino acid, as a result, introduces diverse physicochemical and biological properties in order to be used as a tool to explore protein structure and function or to create novel or enhanced protein for practical purposes.

Diversity

The orthogonal pairs of synthase and tRNA which work for one organism may not work for another as the synthase may mis-aminoacylate endogenous tRNAs or the tRNA be mis-aminoacylated itself by an endogenous synthase. As a result the sets created to date different between organisms.

Orthogonal Sets in E. Coli

- tRNA-TyrRS pair from the archaeon *Methanococcus jannaschii*
- tRNA–LysRS pair from the archaeon *Pyrococcus horikoshii*
- tRNA–GluRS pair from *Methanosarcina mazei*
- leucyl-tRNA synthetase from *Methanobacterium thermoautotrophicum* and a mutant leucyl tRNA derived from *Halobacterium* sp.

Orthogonal Sets in Yeast

- tRNA-TyrRS pair from *Escherichia coli*
- tRNA–LeuRS pair from *Escherichia coli*
- tRNA from human and GlnRS from *Escherichia coli.*

Orthogonal Sets in Mammalian Cells

- tRNA-TyrRS pair from *Bacillus stearothermophilus*
- modified tRNA-TrpRS pair from *Bacillus subtilis* trp
- tRNA–LeuRS pair from *Escherichia coli.*

Protein Studies

With an expanded genetic code, the unnatural amino acid can be genetically directed to any chosen site in the protein of interest.

The high efficiency and fidelity allows a better control of the placement of the modification compared to modifying the protein post-translationally, which generally will target all amino acids of the same type, such as the thiol group of cysteine and the -amino group of lysine. Also, an expanded genetic code allows modifications to be carried out *in vivo*. The ability to site-specifically direct lab-synthesized chemical moieties into proteins allows many types of studies which would otherwise be extremely difficult.

- Probing Protein Structure and Function: by using amino acids with slightly different size such as o-Methyltyrosine or dansylalanine instead of tyrosine, and by inserting genetically-coded reporter moieties (color-changing and/or spin-active) into selected protein sites, chemical information about the protein's structure and function can be measured.
- Identifying and Regulating Protein Activity: by using photocaged aminoacids, protein function can be "switched" on or off by illuminating the organism.
- Changing the mode of action of a protein: one can start with the gene for a protein which binds a certain sequence of DNA, and, by inserting a chemically active amino acid into the binding site, convert it to a protein which cuts the DNA, rather than binding it.
- Improving immunogenicity and overcoming self-tolerance: by replacing strategically-chosen tyrosines with *p*-nitro phenylalanine, a tolerated self-protein can be made immunogenic.

An example of the possible application for this method is the biomedical where "chemical warheads" can be added to protein which target specific cellular components.

Since 2001, 40 non-natural amino acids have been added into protein by creating a unique codon (recoding) and a corresponding transfer-RNA:aminoacyl – tRNA-synthetase pair to encode it with diverse physicochemical and biological properties in order to be used as a tool to exploring protein structure and function or to create novel or enhanced proteins.

Theories on the Origin of the Genetic Code

Despite the minor variations that exist, the genetic code used by all known forms of life is nearly universal. However, there are a huge number of possible genetic codes. If amino acids are randomly associated with triplet codons, there will be 1.5 x 10 possible genetic codes. The question arises: why this code? How did it originate?

Phylogenetic analysis of transfer RNA suggests that tRNA molecules evolved before the present set of aminoacyl-tRNA synthetases.

Theoretically the genetic code could be completely random (a "frozen accident"), completely non-random (optimal) or a combination of random and nonrandom. There are sufficient data to refute the first possibility. For a start, a quick view on the table of the genetic code already shows a clustering of amino acid assignments.

Furthermore, amino acids that share the same biosynthetic pathway tend to have the same first base in their codons, and amino acids with similar physical properties tend to have similar codons. There are four themes running through the many theories that seek to explain the evolution of the genetic code (and hence the origin of these patterns):

- Chemical principles govern specific RNA interaction with amino acids. Aptamer experiments showed that some amino acids have a selective chemical affinity for the base triplets that code for them. Recent experiments show that of the 8 amino acids tested, 6 show some RNA triplet-amino acid association. This has been called the stereochemical code. The stereochemical code could have created an ancient core of assignments. The current complex translation mechanism involving tRNA and associated enzymes may be a later development, and that originally, protein sequences were directly templated on base sequences.

- Biosynthetic expansion. The standard modern genetic code grew from a simpler earlier code through a process of "biosynthetic expansion". Here the idea is that primordial life "discovered" new amino acids (e.g., as by-products of metabolism) and later back-incorporated some of these into the machinery of genetic coding. Although much circumstantial evidence has been found to suggest that fewer different amino acids were used in the past than today, precise and detailed hypotheses about exactly which amino acids entered the code in exactly what order have proved far more controversial.
- Natural selection has led to codon assignments of the genetic code that minimize the effects of mutations. A recent hypothesis suggests that the triplet code was derived from codes that used longer than triplet codons. Longer than triplet decoding has higher degree of codon redundancy and is more error resistant than the triplet decoding. This feature could allow accurate decoding in the absence of highly complex translational machinery such as the ribosome.
- The biocommunicative approach investigates nucleotide sequences as code, i.e. language-like text, which follows in parallel three (3) kinds of rules: combinatorial (syntactic), context-sensitive (pragmatic) and content-specific (semantic). Natural genome editing from this perspective is competent viral-driven generation and integration of meaningful nucleotide sequences into pre-existing genomic content arrangements and the ability to (re-)combine and (re-)regulate them according to context-dependent (i.e. adaptational) purposes of the host organism.
- Information-theoretic approaches treat the genetic code in terms of an error-prone information channel. The inherent noise in the channel poses the organism with a fundamental question: how to construct a genetic code that can withstand the impact of noise while accurately and efficiently translating information? These "rate-distortion" models suggest that the genetic code originated as a result of the interplay of the three conflicting evolutionary forces: the needs for diverse amino-acids, for error-tolerance and for minimal cost of resources. The code emerges at a coding phase transition when the mapping of codons to amino-acids becomes nonrandom. The emergence of the code is governed by the topology defined by the most probable errors and is related to the map colouring problem.

- Genetic code and Codon populations: In other way, considering the global information level of Universal Genetic Code map, studying the whole Human genome codon populations show that the position of each codon within this table precisely dictates its population. So the Universal Genetic Code Table not only maps codons to amino acids, but serves perhaps as a global checksum matrix at the balance level of the whole genome: frequencies of the 64 codons in the whole human genome scale are a self-similar fractal expansion of the universal genetic code map. This global matrix-like function of Genetic Code table was published in September 2010 by the journal *Interdisciplinary Science* reporting that *Codon populations in single-stranded whole human genome DNA Are fractal and fine-tuned by the Golden Ratio 1.618*. In this paper, Jean-Claude Perez shows that Universal Genetic Code Table kernel governs not only the micro scale (codons i.e amino acids) but the macro scale as well. Particularly, the 6 folding steps of codon populations modeled by the binary divisions of the *Dragon fractal paper folding curve* extend the Chargaff's second rule from the domain of single TCAG nucleotides to the larger domain of codon triplets in the case of the whole Human genome.

Control of Gene Expression in Prokaryotes

Control of gene expression in prokaryotes involves control of "operons".

Operon consists of:

1. promoter - DNA sequence where RNA polymerase (transcription enzyme) binds.
2. operator - DNA sequence where an active repressor protein binds.
3. structural genes - DNA coding for protein (usually several that are functionally related, e.g. enzymes of a metabolic pathway).

Regulatory components (NOT part of the operon):

1. regulatory gene - DNA sequence coding for production of a repressor protein (often located away from operon it regulates).
2. repressor protein - in active form, it binds to operator to prevent transcription of structural genes.

Repressible Operon - ex. tryptophan operon : Repressible operons are usually in the "on" condition, i.e. their gene products are generally required most of the time for cell maintenance, etc. Repressor protein is made in an inactive form (it needs to bind to a corepressor to make it an active repressor which can then bind to operator).

Corepressor is usually an end-product of the metabolic pathway coded by the operon, e.g. tryptophan in our example here. Corepressor must accumulate to high levels before it can bind to inactive repressor and make it active.

Inducible Operon - ex. Lactose Operon

Inducible operons are usually in the "off" condition, i.e. their gene products are only occasionally (or never) needed by the cell.

Repressor protein is made in an active form (capable of binding to operator by itself).

Repressor protein can be inactivated by binding to an inducer (lactose in our example here) which then allows the operon to be activated.

Negative vs. Positive Controls

Above examples simply show operons being turned "on" or "off" at the operator, which represents a form of negative control.

Some operons, when turned "on", do not get transcribed at a rate sufficient to see a noticable effect because the RNA polymerase does not bind to promoter effectively.

These operons can be transcribed at a greatly accelerated rate by making the RNA polymerase binding much more efficient. This requires an activated "helper" for the RNA polymerase binding.

Gene Regulation in Eukaryotes

Developmental Biologists have long been interested in how a complex, multicellular organism is able to arise from a single fertilized egg (zygote), i.e. how cells arising from a common lineage (all arising from the zygote) are able to differentiate into the numerous, complex cell types that make up a multicellular organism.

Since the zygote contains ALL the genes necessary for the development of an organism, how is it that only a limited number of these genes are expressed in certain cells so that a multitude of cell types arise from the zygote, e.g. expression of genes for nerve cells, bone cells, skin cells, etc.

At one time, it was generally believed that progressive determination was caused by groups of cells actually losing most of the zygotes original set of genes until a particular cell type contained only genes for forming that cell type, e.g. a cell that eventually becomes a nerve cell has gradually lost all of the genes of the original zygote except those for nerve cell formation.

Today we know that this is generally not the case, although there are exception.

Mitosis faithfully reproduces the full chromosome complement (and all of their genes) to be equally distributed to the new daughter cells, i.e. the daughter cells retain the total genetic potential of the original zygote, "totipotent cells".

Much experimental evidence now supports this concept of the genetic equivalence of nuclei in a multicellular organism.

Nuclear transplantation experiments performed by Robert Briggs and Thomas King, and John Gurdon showed that cells of early embryos retain full genetic potential of zygote.

F.C. Steward was the first to show that individual cells taken from a mature carrot plant could grow into new carrot plants (clones).

More recently the cloning of "Dolly" the sheep, which was not all that important scientifically except that it showed that it could be done in mammals (humans?).

Regeneration, in both plants and animals, have long supported the concept of totipotent cells or the genetic equivalence of somatic cell nuclei.

Therefore, the fact that a differentiating cell is using only a limited number of the total available genes, the problem becomes a differential activation/inactivation of available genes.

For example, cells that eventually become nerve cells do so by activating only the genes necessary for nerve cell formation and likewise inactivating all other genes.

The ways in which cells control gene expression has become a major focus of biological research in the last half of the 20th Century and with the more recent genetic engineering techniques will continue to be a major focus well into this century.

Most of what we first learned about differential gene activation/inactivation came from work on bacteria, e.g. *Escherichia coli.*

Although these cells do not undergo the complex developmental phenomena associated with multicellular organism, they do require activation and inactivation of genes to maintain their existence, and their relative simplicity lent them very well to early studies of gene control.

Many of the models for gene control in prokaryotes have been used as model systems to initially investigate eukaryotic gene control.

However, as one might suspect, the controls used to regulate euakyotic genes appear to be much more complex and must take into account certain aspects of the eukaryote genome that are non-existent in prokaryotes.

1. Very large number of genes present (30,000+) human genes; although only about 3-5% is being used at any one time; recall that *E. coli* has only about 2500 genes.
2. Most eukaryote DNA does not code for RNA or protein (does not function as "genes").
3. Presence of chromatin and the structural complexity of the chromosome.
4. Compartmentalization of most DNA into a nucleus.
5. Complexity in variety of genes being activated at any one time (recall functionally linked genes into operons in bacteria), etc.

One way of looking at "gene expression" is to consider that a gene is expressed (or "activated") only when the product that the gene codes for is produced and functional, e.g. an "active" enzyme.

Considering this very broad description for "gene activation", the eukaryotic cell possesses numerous places where control could take place. Some of these are, at present, only possibilities while others have good experimental support for their existence.

Potential Levels of Eukaryotic Gene Control

Pretranscriptional Control

The physical form of eukaryotic chromatin may be able to block the availability of genes for transcription by forming chromatin structures that "hide" the DNA from trancription factors and enzymes.

"DNA packing" involved basic proteins called HISTONES (H1, H2A, H2B, H3, H4) and various other chromosomal proteins.

An extreme form of DNA packing occurs when chromosomes condense during Prophase of cell division. Very little, if any, gene activity occurs while mitotic/meiotic chromosomes are formed.

Heterochromatin is chromatin in a highly compacted form that is very low or completely devoid of transcriptional activity. It can occur in chromatin found in the Interphase cell.

The tight coiling might be due to high methylation of the DNA in these areas.

Regardless of the cause of heterochromatin, experimental evidence has shown very little transcriptional activity associciated with these areas.

DNA methylation, in general, is a means of inactivating genes over extended time.

An extreme example of gene inactivation by heterochromatin formation is the Barr body typically found in human females. In this example, an entire chromosome's genes are prevented from being transcribed (activated).

A chromosome may have heterochromatin areas interspersed with less compacted areas called euchromatin, which are thought to be areas where the DNA is more available for transcription.

Even in euchromatin, the DNA is tightly wrapped around nucleosomes formed by histones. To make this DNA available for transcription, the histones of the nucleosome appear to undergo acetylation (addition of acetyl groups) which causes a "relaxation" of the DNA/nucleosome association.

This relaxing of the DNA/nucleosome assoication makes the DNA more available for transciption.

Transcriptional Control

Regulatory proteins have also been shown to exist in eukaryotes and may be either activators or repressors of gene activity.

Since the majority of the eukaryotic genes are inactive at any one time, it is believed that most regulators are activators.

Enhancers have also been shown to exist in eukaryotes. These are small stretches of DNA that have the ability to enhance transcriptional activity after binding activator proteins and then interacting at the promoter region to enhance RNA polymerase binding and activity.

Recall that transcription factors are also needed for RNA polymerase binding and activity.

Enhancers are found some distance away from the promoter and may be "upstream" or "downstream" from the promoter.

Posttranscriptional Control

The initial transcript (RNA) in eukaryotes is not functional but must undergo modification to become functional.

rRNA, tRNA, and mRNA must all undergo varying degrees of posttranscriptional modification before they can become functional.

In general, these modifications may include:

1. the cutting out of functional pieces of RNA from a much larger nonfunctional transcript.
2. some of the above pieces may be functional but some require the bonding together of excised pieces to form a single functional piece (exons/introns).
3. mRNA requires the most extensive posttranscriptional modifications, which in addition to the above, require chemical modifications at both ends of the molecule. These modifications may help the transport out of the nucleus, protect the molecule from nuclease attack in the cytoplasm, or somehow be required for initiation of translation.

mRNA is generally consider a "short-lived" molecule in both prokaryotes and eukaryotes, and was once used as a prime criterion for proving that a RNA was in fact a mRNA.

However, exceptions to this generality have been shown in eukaryotes, particularly in certain highly specialized cells (e.g. maturing vertebrate erythrocytes) and developing embryos.

In the case of the maturing vertebrate red blood cell (called erythropoiesis), the erythroblast is a nucleated cell that gradually shuts down most of it's genes except for mRNA for globin production. Huge amounts of globin mRNA accumulate and eventually the cell becomes anucleate, however, the globin mRNA remains for a considerable time afterwards while the cell makes and accumulates very large amounts of hemoglobin.

Unfertilized eggs have been shown to manufacture and accumulate large amounts of mRNA coding for proteins necessary for the rapid, early development of the embryo; these mRNAs are stored in an inactive form in the egg. Activation of the egg, by sperm or artificial means, activates these mRNAs for embryo protein production.

Translational Control

The observation that eggs may contain "long-lived" mRNA but that this RNA is not translated until egg activation has been shown to be a block at translation. A certain initiation factor(s) necessary for translation rapidly becomes available after fertilization (activation).

Also, the amount of heme remaining in maturing red blood cells helps determine how much more globin will be made (translation of globin mRNA).

The poliovirus is thought to select the translation of its "uncapped" mRNAs by somehow destroying the host cell's cap recognition system on the ribosome complex.

Posttranslational Control

Even after the protein is first made, it is not necessarily functional.

Insulin is initially made as a single protein (inactive proinsulin) which must fold back upon itself, form three disulfide bonds, and finally have a small stretch of amino acids removed by a peptidase before it becomes active insulin consisting of two polypeptides held together by two of the disulfide bonds.

Many of the digestive enzymes of the small intestine are synthesized as zymogens (inactive forms) that must undergo enzymatic cleavage to become active, e.g. trypsinogen/trypsin, chymotrypsinogen/chymotrypsin, pepsinogen/pepsin.

Some proteins (malformed, no longer needed, etc.) are "marked" for degradation by proteosomes.

Eukaryotic Gene Organization and its Evolution

Unlike the prokaryotes, eukaryotes do not possesss an "operon type" arrangement of functionally related genes. (recall prokaryote operon).

Instead, it has been shown that genes coding for functionally related products, e.g. a series of enzymes in a metabolic pathway, are scattered throughout the genome and each controlled by a separate promoter, etc.

This gene arrangement may at first appear disorganized but the reality is that it allows much greater variety in the use of these "scattered" genes. Genes can be activated in numerous combinations.

A multigene family is a collection of genes within a genome that are similar or identical in sequence.

The 28S, 18S and 5.8S rRNA genes occur in eukaryotes as tandem arrays of several hundred to several thousand located in association with a nucleosome found inside the nucleus.

The family of globin genes are sequence related but not identical and function in making different hemoglobins at different developmental stages.

Both types of multigene families most likely arose by gene duplication and mutation.

Molecular Biology of Cancer

Cancer is caused by inapproriate gene activity associated with the cell cycle.

Some chararcteristics of malignant cancers (solid types):

1. Loss of cell cycle control
2. Cell surface alterations
3. Secretion of distinct products, e.g. proteolytic enzymes, embryonic antigens, angiogenin, etc.
4. Morphological alterations, enlarged nuclei, aberrant nucleoli, numerous microvilli
5. Highly vascularized
6. Metastasis (travel to distant tissues and establish secondary or "metastatic" cancers).

The genetic basis of cancer was first discovered through the work with retroviruses that were shown to cause cancer in monkeys, chickens, mice, etc.

The viral genes were identified that could be directly linked to the cause of cancer in experimental animals.

These genes were called oncogenes ("cancer genes").

Upon closer examination, researchers found that in fact the oncogenes were not unique but were in fact mutated forms of normal genes (proto-oncogene) found in eukaryotic organisms; including humans.

These normal genes, for the most part, are involved with some aspect of regulating the cell cycle.

Three ways for conversion of a proto-oncogene into an oncogene:

1. translocation or transposition to new promoter
2. gene amplification
3. point mutation within gene.

In addition to proto-oncogenes that can become oncogenes, there are normal, tumour-suppressor genes that are mutated during the formation of cancers.

Tumour-suppressor genes produce products that normally block the cell cycle; which would normally prevent cancers.

The cancerous state results from alteration of several genes, both proto-oncogenes and tumour suppressor genes.

Regulation of Gene Expression in Eukaryotes

The cloning of Dolly, a sheep, was reported worldwide in 1996. Dolly developed from adult somatic nuclei that had been implanted into enucleated eggs (eggs with the nuclei removed). More recently, cows, pigs, mice, and other mammals have been cloned as well with the use of similar technology. The successful cloning of Dolly was a great surprise to the scientific community because the cloning of mammals from somatic cells was thought to be impossible. A reason for the initial skepticism was that the formation of male and female gametes (sperm and egg cells) was known to include sex-specific modifications to the respective genomes that resulted in sex-specific patterns of gene expression. As such, Dolly is symbolic of how far we have progressed in understanding aspects of eukaryotic gene regulation such as the global control of gene expression exemplified by gamete development. However, for every successful clone, including Dolly, there are many more, perhaps hundreds of embryos that fail to develop into viable progeny. The extremely high failure rate underscores how much remains to be deciphered about eukaryotic gene regulation.

The biological properties of each eukaryotic cell type are largely determined by the proteins expressed within it. This constellation of expressed proteins determines much of the cell's architecture, its enzymatic activities, its interactions with its environment, and many other physiological properties. However, at any given time in a cell's life history, only a fraction of the RNAs and proteins encoded in its genome are expressed. At different times, the profile of expressed gene products can differ dramatically, both in regard to which proteins are expressed and at what levels. How are these specific profiles generated?

As one might expect, if the final product is a protein, regulation could be achieved by controlling the transcription of DNA into RNA or the translation of RNA into protein. In fact, gene regulation takes place at many levels, including at the mRNA level (through alterations in splicing or the stability of the mRNA) and after translation (by modifications of proteins). However, most regulation is thought to take place at the level of gene transcription; so, in this chapter, the primary focus is on the regulation of transcription. The basic mechanism at work is that molecular signals from outside or inside the cell lead to the binding of regulatory proteins to specific DNA sites outside of protein-encoding regions, and the binding of these proteins modulates the rate of transcription. These proteins may directly or indirectly assist RNA polymerase in binding to its transcription initiation site—

the *promoter*—or they may repress transcription by preventing the binding of RNA polymerase.

Although bacteria and eukaryotes have much of the logic of gene regulation in common, there are some fundamental differences in the underlying mechanisms and machinery. Both use sequence-specific DNA-binding proteins to modulate the level of transcription. However, eukaryotic genomes are bigger and their range of properties is larger than those of bacteria. Inevitably their regulation is more complex, requiring more types of regulatory proteins and more types of interactionswith the adjacent regulatory regions in DNA. The most important difference is that eukaryotic DNA is packaged into *nucleosomes,* forming *chromatin,* whereas bacterial DNA lacks nucleosomes. In eukaryotes, chromatin structure is dynamic and is an essential ingredient in gene regulation.

In general, the ground state of a bacterial gene is "on." Thus, RNA polymerase can usually bind to a promoter when no other regulatory proteins are around to bind to the DNA. In bacteria, transcription initiation is prevented or reduced if the binding of RNA polymerase is blocked, usually through the binding of a repressor regulatory protein. Activator regulatory proteins increase the binding of RNA polymerase to promoters where a little help is needed. In contrast, the ground state in eukaryotes is "off." Therefore, the transcriptional machinery (including RNA polymerase II and associated general transcription factors) cannot bind to the promoter in the absence of other regulatory proteins. In many cases, the binding of the transcriptional apparatus is not possible, owing to the position of nucleosomes near the promoter. Thus, chromatin structure usually has to be changed to activate eukaryotic transcription. The structure of chromatin around activated or repressed genes within cells can be quite stable and inherited by daughter cells. The inheritance of chromatin structure is a form of inheritance that does not directly entail DNA sequence.

1. In bacteria, all genes are transcribed into RNA by the same RNA polymerase, whereas three RNA polymerases function in eukaryotes.
2. RNA transcripts are extensively processed during transcription in eukaryotes; the 5_ and 3_ ends are modified and introns are spliced out.
3. RNA polymerase II is much larger and more complex than its bacterial counterpart. One reason for the added complexity is

that RNA polymerase II must synthesize RNA *and* coordinate the special processing events unique to eukaryotes.

Multicellular eukaryotes may have as many as 25,000 genes, severalfold more than the average bacterium. Moreover, patterns of eukaryotic gene expression can be extraordinarily complex. That is, there is great variation among genes in when a gene is on (transcribed) or off (not transcribed) and in how much transcript needs to be made. For example, one gene may be transcribed only during early development and another only in the presence of a viral infection. Finally, the majority of the genes in a eukaryotic cell are off at any one time. On the basis of these considerations alone, eukaryotic gene regulation must be able to ensure that the expression of most genes in the genome is off at any one time while activating a subset of genes; and generate thousands of patterns of gene expression.

Mechanisms have evolved to ensure that most of the genes in a eukaryotic cell are not transcribed. Before considering how genes are kept transcriptionally inactive, we will focus on the second point: How are eukaryotic genes able to exhibit an enormous number and diversity of expression patterns? The machinery required for generating so many patterns of gene transcription in vivo has many components, including both regulatory proteins and cis-acting regulatory sequences. To initiate transcription, these proteins interact with DNA sequences called promoter-proximal elements near the promoter of a gene. The second group of protein components consists of specific transcription factors that bind to cis-acting regulatory sequences in the DNA called enhancers or upstream activating sequences (UAS's). These regulatory sequences may be located a considerable distance from gene promoters. Generally speaking, promoters and promoter-proximal elements are bound by transcription factors that affect the expression of many genes. Enhancers are the targets of more specific transcription factors that control the regulation of smaller subsets of genes. Often, an enhancer will act in only one or a few cell types in a multicellular eukaryote.

For RNA polymerase II to transcribe DNA into RNA at a maximum rate, multiple cis-acting regulatory elements must play a part. The promoters, promoter-proximal elements,and enhancers are all targets for binding by different trans-acting DNA binding proteins. The binding of RNA polymerase II to the promoter does not produce efficient transcription by itself.

Transcription requires the binding of general transcription factors to additional promoter-proximal elements that are commonly found within 100 bp of the transcription initiation site of many (but not all) genes. One of these elements is the CCAAT box, and often another is a GC-rich segment farther upstream. The general transcription factors that bind to the promoter-proximal elements are expressed in most cells, and sothey are available to initiate transcription at any time. Mutations in these sites can have a dramatic effect on transcription, demonstrating how important they are.

To modulate transcription, regulatory proteins possess one or more of the following functional domains:

1. A domain that recognizes a DNA regulatory sequence (the protein's DNA-binding site)
2. A domain that interacts with one or more proteins of the transcriptional apparatus (RNA polymerase or a protein associated with RNA polymerase)
3. A domain that interacts with proteins bound to nearby regulatory sequences on DNA such that they can act cooperatively to regulate transcription
4. A domain that influences chromatin condensation either directly or indirectly
5. A domain that acts as a sensor of physiological conditions within the cell Much of the strategy of eukaryotic transcriptional control hinges on how specific transcription factors control the access of general transcription factors and RNA polymerase II. Eukaryotic gene regulatory mechanisms have been discovered through both biochemical and genetic approaches. The latter has been advanced in particular by studies of the single-celled yeast *Saccharomyces cerevisiae.* Several decades of research have been a source of many insights into general principles of how eukaryotic transcriptional regulatory proteins work and how different cell types are generated. We'll examine two yeast gene regulatory systems in detail: the first concerns the galactose-utilization pathway; the second is the control of mating type.

Model Organism *Yeast*

Saccharomyces cerevisiae, or budding yeast, has emerged in recent years as the premier eukaryotic genetic system. Humans have grown yeast for centuries because it is an essential component of beer, bread, and wine. Yeast has many features that make it an ideal model organism. As a unicellular eukaryote, it can be grown on agar plates and, with a life cycle of just 90 minutes, large quantities can be cultured in liquid media. It has a very compact genome with only about 12 megabase pairs of DNA (compared with almost 3000 megabase pairs for humans) containing approximately 6000 genes that are distributed on 16 chromosomes. It was the first eukaryote to have its genome sequenced.

The yeast life cycle makes it very versatile for laboratory studies. Cells can be grown as either diploid or haploid. In both cases, the mother cell produces a bud containing an identical daughter cell. Diploid cells either continue to grow by budding or are induced to undergo meiosis, which produces four haploid spores held together in an *ascus* (also called a *tetrad*). Haploid spores of opposite mating type (a or ‘) will fuse and form a diploid. Spores of the same mating type will continue growth by budding.

Yeast has been called the *E. coli* of eukaryotes because of the ease of forward and reverse mutant analysis. To isolate mutants by using a forward genetic approach, haploid cells are mutagenized (with X rays, for example) and screened on plates for mutant phenotypes. This procedure is usually done by first plating cells on a rich medium on which all cells grow and by copying, or *replica plating,* the colonies from this master plate onto replica plates containing selective media or special growth conditions. For example, temperature-sensitive mutants will grow on the master plate at the permissive temperature but not on a replica plate at a restrictive temperature.

Comparison of the colonies on the master and replica plates will reveal the temperature-sensitive mutants. Using reverse genetics, scientists can also replace any yeast gene (of known or unknown function) with a mutant version (synthesized in a test tube) to understand the nature of the gene product.

Lessons from Yeast: The GAL System

To make use of extracellular galactose, yeast imports the sugar and converts it into a form of glucose that can be metabolized. Several genes—*GAL1, GAL2, GAL7,* and *GAL10*—in the yeast genome encode enzymes that catalyze steps in the biochemical pathway that converts galactose into glucose.

Three additional genes—*GAL3, GAL4,* and *GAL80*—encode proteins that regulate the expression of the enzyme genes. Just as in the *lac* system, the abundance of the sugar determines the level of gene expression in the biochemical pathway. In yeast cells growing in media lacking galactose, the *GAL* genes are largely silent. But, in the presence of galactose (and the absence of glucose), the *GAL* genes are induced. Just as for the *lac* operon, genetic and molecular analyses of mutants have been key to understanding how the expression of the genes in the galactose pathway is controlled.

The key regulator of *GAL* gene expression is the Gal4 protein, a sequencespecific DNA-binding protein. Gal4 is perhaps the best-studied transcriptional regulatory protein in eukaryotes. The detailed dissection of its regulation and activity has been a source of several key insights into the control of transcription in eukaryotes.

Gal4 Regulates Multiple Genes through Upstream Activating Sequences

In the presence of galactose, the *GAL1, GAL2, GAL7,* and *GAL10* genes are induced 1000-fold or more. In *GAL4* mutants, however, they remain silent. Each of these four genes has two or more Gal4-binding sites located 5_ (upstream) of its promoter. Consider the *GAL10* and *GAL1* genes, which are adjacent to each other and transcribed in opposite directions. Between the *GAL1* transcription start site and the *GAL10* transcription start site is a single 118-bp region that contains four Gal4- binding sites. Each Gal4-binding site is 17 base pairs long and is bound by one Gal4 protein dimer. There are two Gal4-binding sites upstream of the *GAL2* gene as well, and another two upstream of the *GAL7* gene. These binding sites are required for gene activation in vivo. If they are deleted, the genes are silent, even in the presence of galactose. These regulatory sequences are enhancers that are also referred to as upstream activating sequences. The presence of enhancers located at a considerable linear distance from a eukaryotic gene's promoter is typical.

The level of gene expression in the biochemical pathway. In yeast cells growing in media lacking galactose, the *GAL* genes are largely silent. But, in the presence of galactose (and the absence of glucose), the *GAL* genes are induced. Just as for the *lac* operon, genetic and molecular analyses of mutants have been key to understanding how the expression of the genes in the galactose pathway is controlled.

The key regulator of *GAL* gene expression is the Gal4 protein, a sequencespecific DNA-binding protein. Gal4 is perhaps the best-studied transcriptional regulatory protein in eukaryotes. The detailed dissection of its regulation and activity has been a source of several key insights into the control of transcription in eukaryotes.

The Gal4 protein has separable DNA-binding and Activation Domains

After Gal4 is bound to the UAS element, how is gene expression induced? A distinct domain of the Gal4 protein, the activation domain, is required for regulatory activity. Thus, the Gal4 protein has at least two domains: one for DNA binding and another for activating transcription. A similar modular organization has been found to be a common feature of other DNA-binding transcription factors as well. The modular organization of the Gal4 protein was demonstrated in a series of simple, elegant experiments. The strategy was to test the DNA binding and gene activation of mutant forms of the protein in which parts had been either deleted or fused to other proteins. In this manner, whether a part of the protein was necessary for a particular function could be determined. To carry out these studies, experimenters needed a simple means of assaying the expression of the enzymes encoded by the *GAL* genes. The expression of *GAL* genes and other targets of transcription factors is typically monitored by using a reporter gene whose expression is easily tracked. Often, the reporter gene is the *lacZ* gene of *E. coli,* which can act on substrates whose products are easily measured by their bright color or fluourescence. Another common reporter gene is the gene that encodes the green fluorescent protein of jellyfish, which, as its name suggests, is easily tracked by the light that it emits. The coding region of one of these reporter genes and a promoter are placed downstream of a UAS element from a *GAL* gene.

Reporter expression is then a read-out of Gal4 activity in cells. When a form of the Gal4 protein lacking the activation domain is expressed in yeast, the binding sites of the UAS element are occupied, but no transcription is stimulated. The same is true when other regulatory proteins lacking activation domains, such as the bacterial repressor LexA, are expressed in cells bearing reporter genes with their respective binding sites. The more interesting result is obtained when a form of the Gal4 protein lacking the DNA-binding domain is grafted to the LexA DNA-binding domain; the hybrid protein now activates transcription from LexAbinding sites. Further "domain swap" experiments have revealed that the transcriptional activation function of the Gal4 protein resides in two small domains about 50 to 100 amino acids in length. These domains are separable from those used in the dimerization of the protein, DNA binding, and interaction with the Gal80 protein. The activation domain helps recruit the transcriptional machinery to the promoter.

This highly modular arrangement of activityregulating domains is found in many transcription factors.

Gal4 Activity is Physiologically Regulated

How does Gal4 become active in the presence of galactose? Key clues came from analyses of mutations in the *GAL80* and *GAL3* genes. In *GAL80* mutants, the *GAL* structural genes are active even in the absence of galactose. This result suggests that the normal function of the Gal80 protein is to somehow inhibit *GAL* gene expression. Conversely, in *GAL3* mutants, the *GAL* structural genes are not active in the presence of galactose, suggesting that Gal3 normally promotes expression of the *GAL* genes.

Extensive biochemical analyses have revealed that the Gal80 protein binds to the Gal4 protein with high affinity and directly inhibits Gal4 activity. Specifically, Gal80 binds to a region within one of the Gal4 activation domains, blocking its ability to promote the transcription of target genes. The role of the Gal3 protein is to release Gal4 from its inhibition by Gal80 in the presence of galactose. Gal3 is a sensor and inducer. When Gal3 binds galactose and ATP, it undergoes an allosteric change that promotes binding to Gal80, which in turn causes Gal80 to release Gal4, which is then able to activate transcription of its target genes. Thus, Gal3, Gal80, and Gal4 are all part of a switch whose state is determined by the presence or absence of galactose. In this switch, DNA binding by the transcriptional regulator is not the physiologically regulated step (as is the case in the *lac* operon and bacteriophage); rather, the activity of the activation domain is regulated.

Gal4 Functions in most Eukaryotes

In addition to its action in yeast cells, Gal4 has been shown to be able to activate transcription in insect cells, human cells, and many other eukaryotic species. This versatility suggests that biochemical machinery and mechanisms of gene activation are common to a broad array of eukaryotes and that features revealed in yeast are generally present in other eukaryotes, and vice versa. Furthermore, because of their versatility, Gal4 and its UAS elements have become favored tools in genetic analysis for manipulating gene expression and function in a wide variety of model systems.

Activators Recruit the Transcriptional Machinery

In bacteria, activators commonly stimulate transcription by interacting directly with DNA and with RNA polymerase. In eukaryotes, activators generally work indirectly to recruit RNA polymerase II to gene promoters through two major mechanisms. First, activators can interact with subunits of the protein complexes having roles in transcription initiation. Second, activators can recruit proteins that modify chromatin structure, allowing RNA polymerase II and other proteins access to the DNA. Many activators, including Gal4, have both activities.

The eukaryotic transcriptional machinery contains many proteins that are parts of various subcomplexes within the transcriptional apparatus that is assembled on gene promoters. One subcomplex, transcription factor IID (TFIID), binds to the TATA box of eukaryotic promoters through the TATAbinding protein. Gal4 binds to TBP at a site in its activation domain, and, through this binding, it recruits the TFIID complex and, in turn, RNA polymerase II to the promoter.

The affinity of this interaction correlates well with Gal4's potency as an activator. Gal4 also interacts with the large Mediator complex, which directly interacts with RNA polymerase II to recruit it to gene promoters. The Mediator complex is an example of a coactivator, a term applied to a protein or protein complex that facilitates gene activation by a transcription factor but that itself is neither part of the transcriptional machinery nor a DNA-binding protein.

The ability of activators to bind to upstream DNA sequences and to interact with proteins that bind directly or indirectly to promoters helps to explain how transcription can be stimulated from more distant regulatory sequences.

Dynamic Chromatin and Eukaryotic Gene Regulation

A second mechanism for influencing gene transcription in eukaryotes modifies the local chromatin structure around gene regulatory sequences. To fully understand how this mechanism works, we need to first review chromatin structure and then consider how it can change and how these changes affect gene expression. The recruitment of transcriptional machinery by activators may appear to be somewhat similar in eukaryotes and bacteria, with the major difference being in the number of interacting proteins in the transcriptional machinery.

Indeed, less than a decade ago, many biologists pictured eukaryotic regulation simply as a biochemically more complicated version of what had been discovered in bacteria. However, this view has changed dramatically as biologists have considered the effect of the organization of genomic DNA in eukaryotes.

Compared with eukaryotic DNA, bacterial DNA is relatively "naked," making it readily accessible to RNA polymerase. In contrast, eukaryotic chromosomes are packaged into chromatin, which is composed of DNA and proteins (mostly histones).

The basic unit of chromatin is the nucleosome, containing about 150 bp of DNA wrapped twice around a histone octamer. The histone octamer is composed of two subunits of each of the four histones: histone 2A, 2B, 3, and 4. Nucleosomes can associate into higherorder structures that further condense the DNA. The packaging of eukaryotic DNA into chromatin means that much of the DNA is not readily accessible to regulatory proteins and the transcriptional apparatus. Thus, whereas prokaryotic genes are generally accessible and "on" unless repressed, eukaryotic genes are inaccessible and "off" unless activated. Therefore, the modification of chromatin structure is a distinctive feature of eukaryotic gene regulation.

One can imagine several ways to alter chromatin structure. For example, one mechanism might be to simply move the histone octamer along the DNA. In the 1980s, biochemical techniques were developed that allowed researchers to determine the position of nucleosomes in and around specific genes. In these studies, chromatin was isolated from tissues or cells in which a gene was on and compared with chromatin from tissue where the same gene was off. The result for most genes analyzed was that nucleosome positions changed, especially in a gene's regulatory regions. Thus, which DNA regions are wrapped up in nucleosomes can change: Nucleosome positions can shift on the DNA from cell to cell and over the life cycle of an organism. Transcription might be repressed when the promoter and flanking sequences are wound up in a nucleosome and inaccessible to RNA polymerase II. Activation of transcription would thus require the blocking nucleosome to be reorganized by nudging the histones or removing them entirely. Conversely, when gene repression is necessary, histone octamers may shift into a position that prevents transcription. The changing of nucleosome position is referred to as chromatin remodeling. Now, chromatin remodeling is known to be an integral part of eukaryotic gene expression, and great advances are being made in determining the underlying mechanism(s) and the regulatory proteins taking part. Here, again, genetic studies in yeast have been pivotal.

Chromatin-remodeling Proteins and Gene Activation

What was the connection between the ability to utilize sugar and the ability to switch mating types? The Snf2–Swi2 protein was purified and discovered to be part of a large, multisubunit complex called the SWI–SNF complex that can reposition nucleosomes in a test-tube assay if ATP is provided as an energy source. In some situations, the multisubunit SWI–SNF complex activates transcription by moving nucleosomes that are covering the TATA sequences and, in this way, facilitates the binding of RNA polymerase II. The SWI–SNF complex is thus a coactivator.

Gal4 also binds to the SWI–SNF complex and recruits the chromatin-remodeling complex to activated promoters. Yeast strains containing a defective SWI–SNF complex show a reduced level of Gal4 activity. Why might an activator use multiple activation mechanisms? There are at least two reasons understood at present. The first is that the accessibility of target promoters may change at different stages of the cell cycle or in different cell types (in multicellular eukaryotes). For example, during mitosis, when chromatin is more condensed, genes are less accessible. At that stage, Gal4 must recruit the chromatin-remodeling complexes, whereas, at other times, such recruitment might not be required to activate gene expression.

A second reason is that many transcription factors act in combinations to control gene expression synergistically. We will see shortly that this combinatorial synergy is a result of the fact that chromatin-remodeling complexes and the transcriptional machinery are recruited more efficiently when multiple transcription factors act together.

Histones and Chromatin Remodeling

A histone code As already stated, most nucleosomes are composed of an octamer made up of two copies each of the four core histones. Histones are known to be the most conserved proteins in nature; that is, histones are almost identical in all eukaryotic organisms from yeast to plants to animals. This conservation contributed to the view that histones could not take part in anything more complicated than the packaging of DNA to fit in the nucleus. However, recall that DNA with its four bases also was considered too "dumb" a molecule to carry the blueprint for all organisms on Earth.

Of note is that the histone proteins are organized into the core octamer with their amino-terminal ends protruding from the nucleosome. These protruding ends are called histone tails. Since the early 1960s, specific lysine residues in the histone tails have been known to be able to be covalently modified by the attachment of acetyl and methyl groups.

These reactions take place after the histone protein has been translated and even after the histone has been incorporated into a nucleosome.

There are now known to be at least 150 different histone modifications that require a wide variety of molecules in addition to the acetyl and methyl groups already mentioned (for example, phosphorylation and ubiquitylation).

Histone acetylation, deacetylation, and gene expression The acetylation reaction is the best-characterized histone modification:

Note that the reaction is reversible, which means that acetyl groups can be added and removed from the same histone residue. With 44 histone lysine residues available to accept acetyl groups, the presence or absence of these groups can carry a tremendous amount of information. For this reason, the covalent modification of histone tails is said to be a histone code. Scientists coined the expression histone code because the covalent modification of histone tails is reminiscent of the genetic code. For the histone code, information is stored in the patterns of histone modification rather than in the sequence of nucleotides. With more than 150 known histone modifications, there are a huge number of possible patterns and their effects on chromatin structure and transcriptional regulation are just beginning to be deciphered. To add to this complexity, the code is likely not interpreted in precisely the same way in all organisms. For now, let's see how the acetylation of histone amino acids influences chromatin structure and gene expression.

Evidence had been accumulating for years that the histones associated with the nucleosomes of active genes are rich in acetyl groups (said to be hyperacetylated), whereas inactive genes are underacetylated (hypoacetylated). The enzyme responsible for adding acetyl groups, histone acetyltransferase (HAT), proved very difficult to isolate. When it was finally isolated and its protein sequence deduced, it was found to be an *ortholog* of a yeast transcriptional activator called GCN5 (meaning that it was encoded by the same gene in a different organism). Thus, the conclusion was that GCN5 is a histone acetyltransferase. It binds to the DNA in the regulatory regions of some genes and activates transcription by acetylating nearby histones. Various protein complexes that are recruited by transcriptional activators are now understood to possess a HAT activity.

How does histone acetylation facilitate changes in gene expression? There appear to be at least two mechanisms for doing so. First, the addition of acetyl groups to specific histone residues can alter the interaction in a nucleosome between the DNA and a histone octamer so that the octamer is more likely to slide along the DNA to a new position. Second, histone acetylation, in conjunction with other histone modifications, influences the binding of regulatory proteins to the DNA. The bound regulatory protein may take part in one of several functions that either directly or indirectly increase the frequency of transcription initiation.

Like other histone modifications, acetylation is reversible, and histone deacetylases (HDAT's) also have been identified.

Such proteins play key roles in gene repression. For example, in the presence of galactose and glucose, the activation of *GAL* genes is prevented by the Mig1 protein. Mig1 is a sequence-specific DNA-binding repressor that binds to a site between the UAS element and the promoter of the *GAL1* gene. Mig1 recruits a protein complex called Tup1 that contains a histone deacetylase and that represses gene transcription. The Tup1 complex is an example of a corepressor, which faciliates gene repression but is not itself a DNA-binding repressor. The Tup1 complex is also recruited by other yeast repressors, such as MAT?2, and counterparts of this complex are found in all eukaryotes.

Mechanism of Enhancer Action

The development of a complex organism requires that transcription levels be regulated over a wide range. Think of a regulation mechanism as more like a rheostat than an on-or-off switch. In eukaryotes, transcription levels are made finely adjustable by the clustering of binding sites into enhancers. Several different transcription factors or several molecules of the same transcription factor may bind to adjacent sites. The binding of these factors to sites that are the correct distance apart leads to an amplified, or superadditive, effect on activating transcription. When an effect is greater than additive, it is said to be synergistic.

The binding of multiple regulatory proteins to the multiple binding sites in an enhancer can catalyze the formation of an enhanceosome, a large protein complex that acts synergistically to activate transcription.

To better understand what an enhanceosome is and how it acts synergistically, let's look at a specific example.

The a-interferon Enhanceosome

The human -interferon gene, which encodes the antiviral protein interferon, is one of the best-characterized genes in eukaryotes. It is normally switched off but is activated to very high levels of transcription on viral infection. The key to the activation of this gene is the assembly of transcription factors into an enhanceosome about 100 bp upstream of the TATA box and transcription start site. The regulatory proteins of the -interferon enhanceosome all bind to the same face of the DNA double helix. Binding to the other side of the helix are several architectural proteins that bend the DNA and allow the different regulatory proteins to touch one another and form an activated complex. When all of the regulatory proteins are bound and interacting correctly, they form a "landing pad," a highaffinity binding site for the protein CBP, a coactivator protein that also recruits the transcriptional machinery. The large CBP protein also contains an intrinsic histone acetylase activity that modifies nucleosomes and facilitates high levels of transcription.

Cooperative interactions help to explain several perplexing observations about enhancers. For example, they explain why mutating any one transcription factor or binding site dramatically reduces enhancer activity. They also explain why the distance between binding sites within the enhancer is such a critical feature. Furthermore, enhancers do not have to be close to the start site of transcription.

The Control of Yeast Mating Type: Combinatorial Interactions

Thus far, we have focused in this chapter on the regulation of single genes or a few genes in one pathway. In multicellular organisms, distinct cell types differ in the expression of hundreds of genes. The expression or repression of sets of genes must therefore be coordinated in the making of particular cell types. One of the best-understood examples of cell-type regulation in eukaryotes is the regulation of mating type in yeast. This regulatory system has been dissected by an elegant combination of genetics, molecular biology, and biochemistry. Mating type serves as an excellent model for understanding the logic of gene regulation in multicellular animals.

The yeast *Saccharomyces cerevisiae* can exist in any of three different cell types known as a, and 'a/'.

The two cell types a and ' are haploid and contain only one copy of each chromosome. Although the two haploid cell types cannot be distinguished by their appearance in the microscope, they can be differentiated by a number of specific cellular characteristics, principally their mating type.

An cell mates only with an a cell and secretes an oligopeptide pheromone, or sex hormone, called factor that arrests a cells in the cell cycle. A cell of the a type mates only with an cell and secretes a pheromone, called a factor, that arrests cells.

The diploid a cell does not mate, is larger than the and a cells, and does not respond to the mating hormones. Genetic analysis of mutants defective in mating has shown that cell type is controlled by a single genetic locus, the mating-type locus, *MAT*. There are two alleles of the *MAT* locus: haploid a cells have the *MATa* allele, haploid ‘ cells have the *MATa* allele, and the a/‘ diploid has both alleles. Although mating type is under genetic control, certain strains switch their mating type, sometimes as frequently as every cell division.

Enhancer-blocking Insulators

A regulatory element, such as an enhancer, that can act over tens of thousands of base pairs could interfere with the regulation of nearby genes. To prevent such promiscuous activation, regulatory elements called enhancer-blocking insulators have evolved. When positioned between an enhancer and a promoter, enhancerblocking insulators prevent the enhancer from activating transcription at that promoter. Such insulators have no effect on the activation of other promoters that are not separated from their enhancers by the insulator. Several models have been proposed to explain how an insulator could block enhancer activity only when placed between an enhancer and a promoter.

Genomic Imprinting

The phenomenon of genomic imprinting was discovered almost 20 years ago in mammals. In genomic imprinting, certain autosomal genes have unusual inheritance patterns. For example, an *igf2* allele is expressed in a mouse only if it is inherited from the mouse's father—an example of maternal imprinting because a copy of the gene derived from the mother is inactive. Conversely, a mouse *H19* allele is expressed only if it is inherited from the mother; *H19* is an example of paternal imprinting because the paternal copy is inactive. The consequence of parental imprinting is that imprinted genes are expressed as if there were only one copy of the gene present in the cell even though there are two. Hence, imprinting is an example of monoallelic inheritance. Importantly, no changes are observed in the DNA sequences of imprinted genes; that is, the identical gene can be active or inactive in the progeny, depending on whether it was inherited from mom or dad.

If the DNA sequence of the gene does not correlate with activity, what does? The answer is that, that the DNA in the regulatory regions of imprinted genes is methylated in a sex-specific manner in the development of gametes. DNA methylation usually results from the enzymatic addition of methyl groups to the carbon-5 position of a specific cytosine residue.

Both DNA methylation marks and histone modification marks can be stably inheritable from one cell generation to the next. We will see later in the chapter how such marks are thought to be duplicated in the course of DNA replication. For now, suffice it to say that such heritable alteration, in which the DNA sequence itself is unchanged, is called epigenetic inheritance, and the alterations (including both DNA methylation and histone modifications) are called epigenetic marks.

Let's turn again to the mouse *ifg2* and *H19* genes to see how imprinting works at the molecular level. These two genes are located in a cluster of imprinted genes on mouse chromosome 7. There are an estimated 100 imprinted genes in the mouse, and most are found in clusters comprising from 3 to 11 imprinted genes. (Humans have most of the same clustered imprintedgenes as those in the mouse.) In all cases examined, there is a specific DNA methylation pattern for each gene copy of an imprinted gene. For the *ifg2–H19* cluster, a specific region of DNA lying between the two genes is methylated in male germ cells and unmethylated in female germ cells. This region is called the imprinting control region (ICR). Only the unmethylated (female) ICR can bind a regulatory protein called CTCF. When bound, CTCF acts as an enhancer-blocking insulator that prevents enhancer activation of *Igf2* transcription. However, the enhancer in females can still activate *H19* transcription. In males, CTCF cannot bind to the ICR and the enhancer can activate *Igf2* transcription (recall that enhancers can act at great distances). The enhancer cannot activate *H19,* however, because the methylated region extends into the *H19* promoter. The methylated promoter cannot bind proteins needed for the transcription of *H19.*

Thus, we see how an enhancer-blocking insulator (in this case, CTCF bound to part of the ICR) prevents the enhancer from activating a distant gene (in this case, *Igf2*). Furthermore, we see that the CTCF-binding site is methylated only in chromosomes derived from the male parent. The methylation of the CTCF-binding site prevents CTCF binding in males and permits the enhancer to activate *Igf2.* Note that parental imprinting can greatly affect pedigree analysis. Because the inherited allele from one parent is inactive, a mutation in the allele inherited from the other parent will appear to be dominant, whereas, in fact, the allele is expressed because only one of the two homologs is active for this gene.

Many steps are required for imprinting. Soon after fertilization, mammals set aside cells that will become their germ cells. Imprints are removed or erased before the germ cells form. Without their distinguishing mark of DNA methylation, these genes are now said to be *epigenetically equivalent.* As these primordial germ cells become fully formed gametes, imprinted genes receive the sex-specific mark that will determine whether the gene will be active or silent after fertilization.

But what about Dolly and other Cloned Mammals?

Genomic imprinting leads to what many thought would be a requirement for the participation of male and female germ cells in mammalian embryo development. That is, male and female gametes contain different subsets of imprinted genes so that the embryo will have a full complement of active imprinted genes. Why then are mammals such as Dolly and, more recently, cloned pigs, cats, dogs, and cows that were derived from somatic nuclei able to survive and even flourish? After all, as already noted, the mutation of even a single imprinted gene can be lethal or can lead to serious disease.

At this point, scientists do not understand why the cloning of many mammalian species has been successful. However, despite these successes, cloning is extremely inefficient in all species tested. For most experiments, a successful clone is an exceedingly rare event, requiring hundreds, even thousands, of attempts. One could argue that the failure of most cloned embryos to develop into viable organisms is a testament to the importance of the epigenetic mechanisms of gene regulation in eukaryotes. As such, it illustrates how knowledge of the complete DNA sequence of all genes in an organism is only a first step in understanding how eukaryotic genes are regulated.

Chromatin Domains and Their Inheritance

Thus far, we have looked at how genes are activated in a chromatin environment. However, as stated at the beginning of this chapter, most of the genes in eukaryotic genomes are off at any one time. Let's now turn to those vast regions of the genome that are transcriptionally inactive. One of the most useful models for understanding mechanisms that maintain the inactivity of genes concerns the control of yeast mating type and mating-type switching.

Mating-type Switching and Gene Silencing

Haploid yeast cells are able to switch their mating type. Genetic analyses of certain mutants that either could not switch or could not mate (they were sterile) were sources of key insights into mating-type switching. Among the switch mutants were several mutant loci including the *HO* gene and the *HMRa* and *HMLa* genes. Further study revealed that the *HO* gene encodes an endonuclease, an enzyme that cleaves DNA, required for the initiation of switching. It was also found that the *HMRa* and *HMLa* loci contain "cassettes" of unexpressed genetic information for the MATa and MAT??mating types, respectively. The *HMR* and *HML* loci are thus referred to as "silent" cassettes.

The HO endonuclease initiates the mating-type switch by inserting a doublestrand break at the *MAT* locus. The interconversion of mating type then takes place by a type of recombination between the segment of DNA (a cassette) from one of the two unexpressed loci and the *MAT* locus. The result is the replacement of the old cassette at the *MAT* locus with a new cassette. The resulting mating type is either the MATa or the MAT??type, depending on which cassette is at the *MAT* locus. The inserted cassette is actually copied from the *HML* or *HMR* locus. In this manner, the switch is reversible because the information for the *a* and *a* cassettes is always present at the *HMR* and *HML* loci and never lost. Normally, the *HMR* and *HML* cassettes are "silent." However, in SIR mutants (silent information regulators), silencing is compromised such that both *a* and *a* information is expressed. The resulting mutants are sterile. The Sir2, Sir3, and Sir4 proteins form a complex that plays a key role in gene silencing. Sir2 is a histone deacetylase that facilitates the condensation of chromatin and helps lock up *HMR* and *HML* in chromatin domains that are inaccessible to transcriptional activators. Gene silencing is a very different process from gene repression; silencing is a position effect that depends on the neighborhood in which genetic information is located. You will learn more about position effects later, in the section on positioneffect variegation in the fruit fly *Drosophila melanogaster*.

Heterochromatin and Euchromatin Compared

Let's return to the silent cassettes *HML* and *HMR* to understand why gene silencing is a very different process from gene repression and what is meant by a genomic neighborhood. To do so, it is important to note that chromatin is not uniform over all chromosomes; certain domains of chromosomes are bundled in highly condensed chromatin called heterochromatin. Other domains are packaged in lesscondensed chromatin called euchromatin.

Chromatin condensation also changes in the course of the cell cycle. The chromatin of cells entering mitosis becomes highly condensed as the chromosomes align in preparation for cell division. After cell division, regions forming heterochromatin remain condensed especially around the centromeres and telomeres (called constitutive heterochromatin), whereas the regions forming euchromatin become less condensed. Geneticists first suspected a limited role for the influence of chromatin structure on gene regulation early in the history of genetics. At that time, they noticed that heterochromatic DNA contained few genes, whereas euchromatin was rich in genes. But what is heterochromatin if not genes? Most of the eukaryotic genome is composed of repetitive sequences that do not make protein or structural RNA—sometimes called junk DNA. Thus, the densely packed nucleosomes of heterochromatin were said to form a "closed" structure that was inaccessible to regulatory proteins and inhospitable to gene activity. In contrast, euchromatin, with its more widely spaced nucleosomes, was proposed to assume an "open" structure that permitted transcription. The existence of open and closed regions of chromatin was also suggested as a reason that recombination frequencies are 100- to 1000-fold higher in euchromatin compared with heterochromatin.

Euchromatin, with its more open conformation, was hypothesized to be more accessible to proteins needed for DNA recombination.

Position-effect Variegation in *Drosophila* Reveals Genomic Neighborhoods

The geneticist Hermann Muller first discovered an interesting genetic phenomenon while studying *Drosophila:* there exist chromosomal neighborhoods that can silence genes that are experimentally "relocated" to adjacent regions of the chromosome.

In these experiments, flies were irradiated with X rays to induce mutations in their germ cells. The progeny of the irradiated flies were screened for unusual phenotypes. A mutation in the *white* gene, near the tip of the X chromosome, will result in progeny with white eyes instead of the wild-type red color. Some of the progeny had very unusual eyes with patches of white and red color. Cytological examination revealed a chromosomal rearrangement in the mutant flies: present in the X chromosome was an inversion of a piece of the chromosome carrying the *white* gene. In this rearrangement, the *white* gene, which is normally located in a euchromatic region of the X chromosome, now finds itself near the heterochromatic centromere.

In some cells, the heterochromatin can "spread" to the neighbouring euchromatin and silences the *white* gene.

Patches of white tissue in the eye are derived from the descendants of a single cell in which the *white* gene has been epigenetically silenced and remains silenced through future cell divisions. In contrast, the red patches arise from cells in which heterochromatin has not spread to the *white* gene, and so this gene remains active in all its descendants. The existence of red and white patches of cells in the eye of a single organism dramatically illustrates two features of epigenetic silencing. First, that the expression of a gene can be repressed by virtue of its position in the chromosome rather than by a mutation in its DNA sequence. Second, that epigenetic silencing can be inherited from one cell generation to the next. Findings from subsequent studies in *Drosophila* and yeast demonstrated that many active genes are silenced in this mosaic fashion when they are relocated to neighborhoods (near centromeres or telomeres) that are heterochromatic. Thus, the ability of heterochromatin to spread into euchromatin and silence genes is a feature common to many organisms. This phenomenon has been called positioneffect variegation (PEV). It provides powerful evidence that chromatin structure is able to regulate the expression of genes—in this case, determining whether genes with identical DNA sequence will be active or silenced.

Genetic Analysis of PEV Reveals Proteins Necessary for Heterochromatin Formation

To find out what proteins might be implicated in the establishment of heterochromatin, geneticists isolated mutations at a second chromosomal locus that either suppressed or enhanced the variegated pattern. Suppressors of variegation [called *Su(var)*] are genes that, when mutated, reduce the spread of heterochromatin, meaning that the wild-type products of these genes are required for spreading. In fact, the *Su(var)* alleles have proved to be a treasure trove for scientists interested in the proteins that are required to establish and maintain the inactive, heterochromatic state.

Among more than 50 *Drosophila* gene products identified by these screens was heterochromatin protein-1 (HP-1), which had previously been found associated with the heterochromatic telomeres and centromeres. Thus, it makes sense that a mutation in the gene encoding HP-1 will show up as a *Su(var)* allele because the protein is required in some way to produce or maintain heterochromatin. Another *Su(var)* gene was found to encode a methyltransferase that adds methyl groups to a specific amino acid residue in the tail of histone H3 (called histone H3 methyltransferase or HMTase).

Proteins similar to HP-1 and HMTase have been isolated in diverse taxa, suggesting the conservation of an important eukaryotic function.

Silencing an Entire Chromosome: X-chromosome Inactivation

The epigenetic phenomenon called X-chromosome inactivation has intrigued scientists for decades. For now, it is sufficient to know that the number of transcripts produced by a gene is usually proportional to the number of copies of that gene in a cell. Mammals, for example, are diploid and have two copies of each gene located on their autosomes. For the vast majority of genes, both alleles are expressed. However, this is not possible for the sex chromosomes.

The number of the X and Y sex chromosomes differs between the sexes, with female mammals having two X chromosomes and males having only one. The mammalian X chromosome is thought to contain about 1000 genes. Females have twice as many copies of these X-linked genes and would otherwise express twice as much transcript from these genes as males do if there were not a mechanism to correct this imbalance. (Not having a Y chromosome is not a problem for females, because the very few genes on this chromosome are required only for the development of males.) This dosage imbalance is corrected by a process called dosage compensation, which makes the amount of most gene products from the two copies of the X chromosome in females equivalent to the single dose of the X chromosome in males.

In mammals, this equivalency is accomplished by random inactivation of one of the two X chromosomes in each cell at an early stage in development. This inactive state is then propagated to all progeny cells. (In the germ line, the second X chromosome becomes reactivated in oogenesis). The inactivated chromosome, called a Barr body, can be seen in the nucleus as a darkly staining, highly condensed, heterochromatic structure. Two aspects of X-chromosome inactivation are relevant to a discussion of chromatin and the regulation of gene expression. First, most of the genes on the inactivated X chromosome are silenced, and the chromosome has epigenetic marks associated with heterochromatin including methylation of H3 at lysine 9 and hypermethylation of its DNA. Second, genes on the inactivated chromosome remain inactive in all descendants of these cells. Because the DNA sequence itself is unchanged, this heritable alteration is an example of epigenetic inheritance.

The Inheritance of Epigenetic Marks and Chromatin Structure

Epigenetic inheritance can be defined operationally as the inheritance of chromatin states from one cell generation to the next. What this inheritance means is that, in DNA replication, both the DNA sequence and the chromatin structure are faithfully passed on to the next cell generation. However, unlike the sequence of DNA, chromatin structure can change in the course of the cell cycle when, for example, transcription factors modify the histone code, causing local changes in nucleosome position or nucleosome density or both.

The replisome not only copies the parental strands but also disassembles the nucleosomes in the parental strands and reassembles them in both the parental and the daughter strands. This process is accomplished by the random distribution of the old histones from existing nucleosomes to daughter strands and the delivery of new histones to the replisome. In this way, the old histones with their modified tails and the new histones with unmodified tails are assembled into nucleosomes that become associated with both daughter strands. The code carried by the old histones most likely guides the modification of the new histones.

The inheritance of DNA methylation is better understood. Semiconservative replication generates daughter helices that are methylated on one of their two strands (the parental strand). The unmethylated strands are methylated by DNA methyltransferases that have a high affinity for these so-called hemimethylated substrates and are guided by the methylation pattern on the parental strand. Thus, the information inherent in the histone code and the existing DNA methylation patterns serve to reconstitute the local chromatin structure that existed before DNA synthesis and mitosis.

Mutations

Mutations are changes in a genomic sequence: the DNA sequence of a cell's genome or the DNA or RNA sequence of a virus. Mutations are caused by radiation, viruses, transposons and mutagenic chemicals, as well as errors that occur during meiosis or DNA replication. They can also be induced by the organism itself, by cellular processes such as hypermutation.

Mutation can result in several different types of change in DNA sequences; these can either have no effect, alter the product of a gene, or prevent the gene from functioning properly or completely. Studies in the fly *Drosophila melanogaster* suggest that if a mutation changes a protein produced by a gene, this will probably be harmful, with about 70 percent of these mutations having damaging effects, and the remainder being either neutral or weakly beneficial. Due to the damaging effects that mutations can have on cells, organisms have evolved mechanisms such as DNA repair to remove mutations. Therefore, the optimal mutation rate for a species is a trade-off between costs of a high mutation rate, such as deleterious mutations, and the metabolic costs of maintaining systems to reduce the mutation rate, such as DNA repair enzymes. Viruses that use RNA as their genetic material have rapid mutation rates, which can be an advantage since these viruses will evolve constantly and rapidly, and thus evade the defensive responses of e.g. the human immune system.

Description

Mutations can involve large sections of DNA becoming duplicated, usually through genetic recombination. These duplications are a major source of raw material for evolving new genes, with tens to hundreds of genes duplicated in animal genomes every million years. Most genes belong to larger families of genes of shared ancestry. Novel genes are produced by several methods, commonly through the duplication and mutation of an ancestral gene, or by recombining parts of different genes to form new combinations with new functions. Here, domains act as modules, each with a particular and independent function, that can be mixed together to produce genes encoding new proteins with novel properties.

For example, the human eye uses four genes to make structures that sense light: three for color vision and one for night vision; all four arose from a single ancestral gene. Another advantage of duplicating a gene (or even an entire genome) is that this increases redundancy; this allows one gene in the pair to acquire a new function while the other copy performs the original function. Other types of mutation occasionally create new genes from previously non-coding DNA.

Changes in chromosome number may involve even larger mutations, where segments of the DNA within chromosomes break and then rearrange. For example, two chromosomes in the *Homo* genus fused to produce human chromosome 2; this fusion did not occur in the lineage of the other apes, and they retain these separate chromosomes. In evolution, the most important role of such chromosomal rearrangements may be to accelerate the divergence of a population into new species by making populations less likely to interbreed, and thereby preserving genetic differences between these populations.

Sequences of DNA that can move about the genome, such as transposons, make up a major fraction of the genetic material of plants and animals, and may have been important in the evolution of genomes. For example, more than a million copies of the Alu sequence are present in the human genome, and these sequences have now been recruited to perform functions such as regulating gene expression. Another effect of these mobile DNA sequences is that when they move within a genome, they can mutate or delete existing genes and thereby produce genetic diversity.

In multicellular organisms with dedicated reproductive cells, mutations can be subdivided into germ line mutations, which can be passed on to descendants through their reproductive cells, and somatic mutations (also called acquired mutations), which involve cells outside the dedicated reproductive group and which are not usually transmitted to descendants. If the organism can reproduce asexually through mechanisms such as cuttings or budding the distinction can become blurred.

For example, plants can sometimes transmit somatic mutations to their descendants asexually or sexually where flower buds develop in somatically mutated parts of plants. A new mutation that was not inherited from either parent is called a *de novo* mutation. The source of the mutation is unrelated to the consequence, although the consequences are related to which cells were mutated.

Nonlethal mutations accumulate within the gene pool and increase the amount of genetic variation. The abundance of some genetic changes within the gene pool can be reduced by natural selection, while other "more favourable" mutations may accumulate and result in adaptive evolutionary changes.

For example, a butterfly may produce offspring with new mutations. The majority of these mutations will have no effect; but one might change the color of one of the butterfly's offspring, making it harder (or easier) for predators to see. If this color change is advantageous, the chance of this butterfly surviving and producing its own offspring are a little better, and over time the number of butterflies with this mutation may form a larger percentage of the population.

Neutral mutations are defined as mutations whose effects do not influence the fitness of an individual. These can accumulate over time due to genetic drift. It is believed that the overwhelming majority of mutations have no significant effect on an organism's fitness. Also,

DNA repair mechanisms are able to mend most changes before they become permanent mutations, and many organisms have mechanisms for eliminating otherwise permanently mutated somatic cells.

Mutation is generally accepted by biologists as the mechanism by which natural selection acts, generating advantageous new traits that survive and multiply in offspring as well as disadvantageous traits, in less fit offspring, that tend to die out.

Causes

Two classes of mutations are spontaneous mutations (molecular decay) and induced mutations caused by mutagens.

Spontaneous mutations on the molecular level can be caused by:

- Tautomerism – A base is changed by the repositioning of a hydrogen atom, altering the hydrogen bonding pattern of that base resulting in incorrect base pairing during replication.
- Depurination – Loss of a purine base (A or G) to form an apurinic site (AP site).
- Deamination – Hydrolysis changes a normal base to an atypical base containing a keto group in place of the original amine group. Examples include C '! U and A '! HX (hypoxanthine), which can be corrected by DNA repair mechanisms; and 5MeC (5-methylcytosine) '! T, which is less likely to be detected as a mutation because thymine is a normal DNA base.
- Slipped strand mispairing - Denaturation of the new strand from the template during replication, followed by renaturation in a different spot ("slipping"). This can lead to insertions or deletions.

Induced mutations on the molecular level can be caused by:

- Chemicals
  - o Hydroxylamine NH_2OH
  - o Base analogs (e.g. BrdU)
  - o Alkylating agents (e.g. *N*-ethyl-*N*-nitrosourea) These agents can mutate both replicating and non-replicating DNA. In contrast, a base analog can only mutate the DNA when the analog is incorporated in replicating the DNA. Each of these classes of chemical mutagens has certain effects that then lead to transitions, transversions, or deletions.
  - o Agents that form DNA adducts (e.g. ochratoxin A metabolites)

- o DNA intercalating agents (e.g. ethidium bromide)
- o DNA crosslinkers
- o Oxidative damage
- o Nitrous acid converts amine groups on A and C to diazo groups, altering their hydrogen bonding patterns which leads to incorrect base pairing during replication.

- Radiation

- o Ultraviolet radiation (nonionizing radiation). Two nucleotide bases in DNA – cytosine and thymine – are most vulnerable to radiation that can change their properties. UV light can induce adjacent pyrimidine bases in a DNA strand to become covalently joined as a pyrimidine dimer. UV radiation, particularly longer-wave UVA, can also cause oxidative damage to DNA.
- o Ionizing radiation

- Viral infections.

DNA has so-called hotspots, where mutations occur up to 100 times more frequently than the normal mutation rate. A hotspot can be at an unusual base, e.g., 5-methylcytosine.

Mutation rates also vary across species. Evolutionary biologists have theorized that higher mutation rates are beneficial in some situations, because they allow organisms to evolve and therefore adapt more quickly to their environments. For example, repeated exposure of bacteria to antibiotics, and selection of resistant mutants, can result in the selection of bacteria that have a much higher mutation rate than the original population (mutator strains).

Classification of Mutation Types

By Effect on Structure

The sequence of a gene can be altered in a number of ways. Gene mutations have varying effects on health depending on where they occur and whether they alter the function of essential proteins. Mutations in the structure of genes can be classified as:

- Small-scale mutations, such as those affecting a small gene in one or a few nucleotides, including:
  - o Point mutations, often caused by chemicals or malfunction of DNA replication, exchange a single nucleotide for another. These changes are classified as transitions or transversions. Most common is the transition that exchanges a purine for

a purine (A ”! G) or a pyrimidine for a pyrimidine, (C ”! T). A transition can be caused by nitrous acid, base mispairing, or mutagenic base analogs such as 5-bromo-2-deoxyuridine (BrdU). Less common is a transversion, which exchanges a purine for a pyrimidine or a pyrimidine for a purine (C/T ”! A/G). An example of a transversion is adenine (A) being converted into a cytosine (C). A point mutation can be reversed by another point mutation, in which the nucleotide is changed back to its original state (true reversion) or by second-site reversion (a complementary mutation elsewhere that results in regained gene functionality). Point mutations that occur within the protein coding region of a gene may be classified into three kinds, depending upon what the erroneous codon codes for:

* Silent mutations: which code for the same amino acid.
* Missense mutations: which code for a different amino acid.
* Nonsense mutations: which code for a stop and can truncate the protein.

o Insertions add one or more extra nucleotides into the DNA. They are usually caused by transposable elements, or errors during replication of repeating elements (e.g. AT repeats). Insertions in the coding region of a gene may alter splicing of the mRNA (splice site mutation), or cause a shift in the reading frame (frameshift), both of which can significantly alter the gene product. Insertions can be reverted by excision of the transposable element.

o Deletions remove one or more nucleotides from the DNA. Like insertions, these mutations can alter the reading frame of the gene. They are generally irreversible: though exactly the same sequence might theoretically be restored by an insertion, transposable elements able to revert a very short deletion (say 1–2 bases) in *any* location are either highly unlikely to exist or do not exist at all. Note that a deletion is not the exact opposite of an insertion: the former is quite random while the latter consists of a specific sequence inserting at locations that are not entirely random or even quite narrowly defined.

- Large-scale mutations in chromosomal structure, including:
  - o Amplifications (or gene duplications) leading to multiple copies of all chromosomal regions, increasing the dosage of the genes located within them.
  - o Deletions of large chromosomal regions, leading to loss of the genes within those regions.
  - o Mutations whose effect is to juxtapose previously separate pieces of DNA, potentially bringing together separate genes to form functionally distinct fusion genes (e.g. bcr-abl). These include:
    - * Chromosomal translocations: interchange of genetic parts from nonhomologous chromosomes.
    - * Interstitial deletions: an intra-chromosomal deletion that removes a segment of DNA from a single chromosome, thereby apposing previously distant genes. For example, cells isolated from a human astrocytoma, a type of brain tumour, were found to have a chromosomal deletion removing sequences between the "fused in glioblastoma" gene and the receptor tyrosine kinase "ros", producing a fusion protein (FIG-ROS). The abnormal FIG-ROS fusion protein has constitutively active kinase activity that causes oncogenic transformation (a transformation from normal cells to cancer cells).
    - * Chromosomal inversions: reversing the orientation of a chromosomal segment.
  - o Loss of heterozygosity: loss of one allele, either by a deletion or recombination event, in an organism that previously had two different alleles.

By Effect on Function

- Loss-of-function mutations are the result of gene product having less or no function. When the allele has a complete loss of function (null allele) it is often called an amorphic mutation. Phenotypes associated with such mutations are most often recessive. Exceptions are when the organism is haploid, or when the reduced dosage of a normal gene product is not enough for a normal phenotype (this is called haploinsufficiency).

- Gain-of-function mutations change the gene product such that it gains a new and abnormal function. These mutations usually have dominant phenotypes. Often called a neomorphic mutation.
- Dominant negative mutations (also called antimorphic mutations) have an altered gene product that acts antagonistically to the wild-type allele. These mutations usually result in an altered molecular function (often inactive) and are characterised by a dominant or semi-dominant phenotype. In humans, Marfan syndrome is an example of a dominant negative mutation occurring in an autosomal dominant disease. In this condition, the defective glycoprotein product of the fibrillin gene (FBN1) antagonizes the product of the normal allele.
- Lethal mutations are mutations that lead to the death of the organisms which carry the mutations.
- A back mutation or reversion is a point mutation that restores the original sequence and hence the original phenotype.

By Effect on Fitness

In applied genetics it is usual to speak of mutations as either harmful or beneficial.

- A harmful mutation is a mutation that decreases the fitness of the organism.
- A beneficial mutation is a mutation that increases fitness of the organism, or which promotes traits that are desirable.

In theoretical population genetics, it is more usual to speak of such mutations as deleterious or advantageous. In the neutral theory of molecular evolution, genetic drift is the basis for most variation at the molecular level.

- A neutral mutation has no harmful or beneficial effect on the organism. Such mutations occur at a steady rate, forming the basis for the molecular clock.
- A deleterious mutation has a negative effect on the phenotype, and thus decreases the fitness of the organism.
- An advantageous mutation has a positive effect on the phenotype, and thus increases the fitness of the organism.
- A nearly neutral mutation is a mutation that may be slightly deleterious or advantageous, although most nearly neutral mutations are slightly deleterious.

In reality, viewing the fitness effects of mutations in these discrete categories is an oversimplification. Attempts have been made to infer the distribution of fitness effects using mutagenesis experiments or theoretical models applied to molecular sequence data.

However, the current distribution is still uncertain, and some aspects of the distribution likely vary between species.

By Inheritance

- inheritable generic in pro-generic tissue or cells on path to be changed to gametes.
- non inheritable somatic (e.g., carcinogenic mutation)
- non inheritable post mortem aDNA mutation in decaying remains.

By pattern of inheritance The human genome contains two copies of each gene – a paternal and a maternal allele.

- A heterozygous mutation is a mutation of only one allele.
- A homozygous mutation is an identical mutation of both the paternal and maternal alleles.
- Compound heterozygous mutations or a genetic compound comprises two different mutations in the paternal and maternal alleles.
- A wildtype or homozygous non-mutated organism is one in which neither allele is mutated. (Just not a mutation).

By Impact on Protein Sequence

- A frameshift mutation is a mutation caused by insertion or deletion of a number of nucleotides that is not evenly divisible by three from a DNA sequence. Due to the triplet nature of gene expression by codons, the insertion or deletion can disrupt the reading frame, or the grouping of the codons, resulting in a completely different translation from the original. The earlier in the sequence the deletion or insertion occurs, the more altered the protein produced is.
- A nonsense mutation is a point mutation in a sequence of DNA that results in a premature stop codon, or a *nonsense codon* in the transcribed mRNA, and possibly a truncated, and often nonfunctional protein product.
- Missense mutations or *nonsynonymous mutations* are types of point mutations where a single nucleotide is changed to cause

substitution of a different amino acid. This in turn can render the resulting protein nonfunctional. Such mutations are responsible for diseases such as Epidermolysis bullosa, sickle-cell disease, and SOD1 mediated ALS (Boillée 2006, p. 39).

- A neutral mutation is a mutation that occurs in an amino acid codon which results in the use of a different, but chemically similar, amino acid. The similarity between the two is enough that little or no change is often rendered in the protein. For example, a change from AAA to AGA will encode lysine, a chemically similar molecule to the intended arginine.
- Silent mutations are mutations that do not result in a change to the amino acid sequence of a protein. They may occur in a region that does not code for a protein, or they may occur within a codon in a manner that does not alter the final amino acid sequence. The phrase *silent mutation* is often used interchangeably with the phrase *synonymous mutation*; however, synonymous mutations are a subcategory of the former, occurring only within exons. The name silent could be a misnomer. For example, a silent mutation in the exon/intron border may lead to alternative splicing by changing the splice site, thereby leading to a changed protein.

Special Classes

- Conditional mutation is a mutation that has wild-type (or less severe) phenotype under certain "permissive" environmental conditions and a mutant phenotype under certain "restrictive" conditions. For example, a temperature-sensitive mutation can cause cell death at high temperature (restrictive condition), but might have no deleterious consequences at a lower temperature (permissive condition).

Nomenclature

Nomenclature of mutations specify the type of mutation and base or amino acid changes.

- Nucleotide substitution (e.g. 76A>T) - The number is the position of the nucleotide from the 5' end, the first letter represents the wild type nucleotide, and the second letter represents the nucleotide which replaced the wild type. In the given example, the adenine at the 76th position was replaced by a thymine.
  - o If it becomes necessary to differentiate between mutations in genomic DNA, mitochondrial DNA, and RNA, a simple

convention is used. For example, if the 100th base of a nucleotide sequence mutated from G to C, then it would be written as g.100G>C if the mutation occurred in genomic DNA, m.100G>C if the mutation occurred in mitochondrial DNA, or r.100g>c if the mutation occurred in RNA. Note that for mutations in RNA, the nucleotide code is written in lower case.

- Amino acid substitution (e.g. D111E) – The first letter is the one letter code of the wild type amino acid, the number is the position of the amino acid from the N terminus, and the second letter is the one letter code of the amino acid present in the mutation. Nonsense mutations are represented with an X for the second amino acid (e.g. D111X).
- Amino acid deletion (e.g. ÄF508) – The Greek letter Ä (delta) indicates a deletion. The letter refers to the amino acid present in the wild type and the number is the position from the N terminus of the amino acid were it to be present as in the wild type.

Harmful Mutations

Changes in DNA caused by mutation can cause errors in protein sequence, creating partially or completely non-functional proteins. To function correctly, each cell depends on thousands of proteins to function in the right places at the right times. When a mutation alters a protein that plays a critical role in the body, a medical condition can result. A condition caused by mutations in one or more genes is called a genetic disorder. Some mutations alter a gene's DNA base sequence but do not change the function of the protein made by the gene. Studies of the fly *Drosophila melanogaster* suggest that if a mutation does change a protein, this will probably be harmful, with about 70 percent of these mutations having damaging effects, and the remainder being either neutral or weakly beneficial. However, studies in yeast have shown that only 7% of mutations that are not in genes are harmful.

If a mutation is present in a germ cell, it can give rise to offspring that carries the mutation in all of its cells. This is the case in hereditary diseases. On the other hand, a mutation may occur in a somatic cell of an organism. Such mutations will be present in all descendants of this cell within the same organism, and certain mutations can cause the cell to become malignant, and thus cause cancer.

Often, gene mutations that could cause a genetic disorder are repaired by the DNA repair system of the cell. Each cell has a number of pathways through which enzymes recognize and repair mistakes in DNA. Because DNA can be damaged or mutated in many ways, the process of DNA repair is an important way in which the body protects itself from disease.

Beneficial Mutations

Although most mutations that change protein sequences are neutral or harmful, some mutations have a positive effect on an organism. In this case, the mutation may enable the mutant organism to withstand particular environmental stresses better than wild-type organisms, or reproduce more quickly.

In these cases a mutation will tend to become more common in a population through natural selection.

For example, a specific 32 base pair deletion in human CCR5 (CCR5-Ä32) confers HIV resistance to homozygotes and delays AIDS onset in heterozygotes. The CCR5 mutation is more common in those of European descent. One possible explanation of the etiology of the relatively high frequency of CCR5-Ä32 in the European population is that it conferred resistance to the bubonic plague in mid-14th century Europe. People with this mutation were more likely to survive infection; thus its frequency in the population increased. This theory could explain why this mutation is not found in southern Africa, where the bubonic plague never reached. A newer theory suggests that the selective pressure on the CCR5 Delta 32 mutation was caused by smallpox instead of the bubonic plague.

Another example, is Sickle cell disease which is a blood disorder in which the body produces an abnormal type of the oxygen-carrying substance hemoglobin in the red blood cells. One-third of all indigenous inhabitants of Sub-Saharan Africa carry the gene, because in areas where malaria is common, there is a survival value in carrying only a single sickle-cell gene (sickle cell trait). Those with only one of the two alleles of the sickle-cell disease are more resistant to malaria, since the infestation of the malaria plasmodium is halted by the sickling of the cells which it infests.

Prion Mutation

Prions are proteins and do not contain genetic material. However, prion replication has been shown to be subject to mutation and natural selection just like other forms of replication.

Cancer

Cancer (medical term: malignant neoplasm) is a class of diseases in which a group of cells display *uncontrolled growth* (division beyond the normal limits), *invasion* (intrusion on and destruction of adjacent tissues), and sometimes *metastasis* (spread to other locations in the body via lymph or blood). These three malignant properties of cancers differentiate them from benign tumors, which are self-limited, and do not invade or metastasize. Most cancers form a tumour but some, like leukemia, do not. The branch of medicine concerned with the study, diagnosis, treatment, and prevention of cancer is oncology. Cancer affects people at all ages with the risk for most types increasing with age. Cancer caused about 13% of all human deaths in 2007 (7.6 million).

Cancers are caused by abnormalities in the genetic material of the transformed cells. These abnormalities may be due to the effects of carcinogens, such as tobacco smoke, radiation, chemicals, or infectious agents. Other cancer-promoting genetic abnormalities may randomly occur through errors in DNA replication, or are inherited, and thus present in all cells from birth. The heritability of cancers is usually affected by complex interactions between carcinogens and the host's genome.

Genetic abnormalities found in cancer typically affect two general classes of genes. Cancer-promoting *oncogenes* are typically activated in cancer cells, giving those cells new properties, such as hyperactive growth and division, protection against programmed cell death, loss of respect for normal tissue boundaries, and the ability to become established in diverse tissue environments. *Tumour suppressor genes* are then inactivated in cancer cells, resulting in the loss of normal functions in those cells, such as accurate DNA replication, control over the cell cycle, orientation and adhesion within tissues, and interaction with protective cells of the immune system.

Definitive diagnosis requires the histologic examination of a biopsy specimen, although the initial indication of malignancy can be symptomatic or radiographic imaging abnormalities. Most cancers can be treated and some forced into remission, depending on the specific type, location, and stage. Once diagnosed, cancer is usually treated with a combination of surgery, chemotherapy and radiotherapy. As research develops, treatments are becoming more specific for different varieties of cancer. There has been significant progress in the development of targeted therapy drugs that act specifically on detectable molecular abnormalities in certain tumors, and which minimize damage to normal cells. The prognosis of cancer patients is most influenced by the type of cancer, as well as the stage, or extent of the disease. In addition, histologic grading and the presence of specific molecular markers can also be useful in establishing prognosis, as well as in determining individual treatments.

Classification

Cancers are classified by the type of cell that resembles the tumour and, therefore, the tissue presumed to be the origin of the tumour. These are the histology and the location, respectively. Examples of general categories include:

- Carcinoma: Malignant tumors derived from epithelial cells. This group represents the most common cancers, including the common forms of breast, prostate, lung and colon cancer.
- Sarcoma: Malignant tumors derived from connective tissue, or mesenchymal cells.
- Lymphoma and leukemia: Malignancies derived from hematopoietic (blood-forming) cells
- Germ cell tumour: Tumors derived from totipotent cells. In adults most often found in the testicle and ovary; in fetuses, babies, and young children most often found on the body midline, particularly at the tip of the tailbone; in horses most often found at the poll (base of the skull).
- Blastic tumour or blastoma: A tumour (usually malignant) which resembles an immature or embryonic tissue. Many of these tumors are most common in children.

Malignant tumors (cancers) are usually named using -carcinoma, -sarcoma or -blastoma as a suffix, with the Latin or Greek word for the organ of origin as the root. For instance, a cancer of the liver is called *hepatocarcinoma*; a cancer of the fat cells is called *liposarcoma*. For common cancers, the English organ name is used. For instance, the most common type of breast cancer is called *ductal carcinoma of the breast* or *mammary ductal carcinoma*. Here, the adjective *ductal* refers to the appearance of the cancer under the microscope, resembling normal breast ducts.

Benign tumors (which are not cancers) are named using -oma as a suffix with the organ name as the root. For instance, a benign tumour of the smooth muscle of the uterus is called *leiomyoma* (the common name of this frequent tumour is *fibroid*). Unfortunately, some cancers also use the -oma suffix, examples being melanoma and seminoma.

Signs and Symptoms

Roughly, cancer symptoms can be divided into three groups:

- *Local symptoms*: unusual lumps or swelling (*tumour*), hemorrhage (bleeding), pain and/or ulceration. Compression of surrounding tissues may cause symptoms such as jaundice (yellowing the eyes and skin).
- *Symptoms of metastasis (spreading)*: enlarged lymph nodes, cough and hemoptysis, hepatomegaly (enlarged liver), bone pain, fracture of affected bones and neurological symptoms. Although advanced cancer may cause pain, it is often not the first symptom.
- *Systemic symptoms*: weight loss, poor appetite, fatigue and cachexia (wasting), excessive sweating (night sweats), anemia and specific paraneoplastic phenomena, i.e. specific conditions that are due to an active cancer, such as thrombosis or hormonal changes.

Every symptom in the above list can be caused by a variety of conditions (a list of which is referred to as the differential diagnosis). Cancer may be a common or uncommon cause of each item.

Causes

Cancer is a diverse class of diseases which differ widely in their causes and biology. Any organism, even plants, can acquire cancer. Nearly all known cancers arise gradually, as errors build up in the cancer cell and its progeny. Anything which replicates (living cells) will probabilistically suffer from errors (mutations). Unless error correction and prevention is properly carried out, the errors will survive, and might be passed along to daughter cells. Normally, the body safeguards against cancer via numerous methods, such as: apoptosis, helper molecules (some DNA polymerases), possibly senescence, etc. However these error-correction methods often fail in small ways, especially in environments that make errors more likely to arise and propagate. For example, such environments can include the presence of disruptive substances called carcinogens, or periodic injury (physical, heat, etc.), or environments that cells did not evolve to withstand, such as hypoxia. Cancer is thus a *progressive* disease, and these progressive errors slowly accumulate until a cell begins to act contrary to its function in the organism.

The errors which cause cancer are often *self-amplifying*, eventually compounding at an exponential rate. For example:

- A mutation in the error-correcting machinery of a cell might cause that cell and its children to accumulate errors more rapidly
- A mutation in signalling (endocrine) machinery of the cell can send error-causing signals to nearby cells
- A mutation might cause cells to become neoplastic, causing them to migrate and disrupt more healthy cells
- Amutation may cause the cell to become immortal, causing them to disrupt healthy cells forever.

Thus cancer often explodes in something akin to a chain reaction caused by a few errors, which compound into more severe errors. Errors which produce more errors are effectively the root cause of cancer, and also the reason that cancer is so hard to treat: even if there were 10,000,000,000 cancerous cells and one killed all but 10 of those cells, those cells (and other error-prone precancerous cells) could still self-replicate or send error-causing signals to other cells, starting the process over again. This rebellion-like scenario is an undesirable survival of the fittest, where the driving forces of evolution work against the body's design and enforcement of order. In fact, once cancer has begun to develop, this same force continues to drive the progression of cancer towards more invasive stages, and is called clonal evolution.

Research about cancer causes often falls into the following categories:

- Agents (e.g. viruses) and events (e.g. mutations) which cause or facilitate genetic changes in cells destined to become cancer.
- The precise nature of the genetic damage, and the genes which are affected by it.
- The consequences of those genetic changes on the biology of the cell, both in generating the defining properties of a cancer cell, and in facilitating additional genetic events which lead to further progression of the cancer.

Chemicals

Cancer pathogenesis is traceable back to DNA mutations that impact cell growth and metastasis. Substances that cause DNA mutations are known as mutagens, and mutagens that cause cancers are known as carcinogens. Particular substances have been linked to specific types of cancer. Tobacco smoking is associated with many forms of cancer, and causes 90% of lung cancer. Prolonged exposure to asbestos fibres is associated with mesothelioma.

Many mutagens are also carcinogens, but some carcinogens are not mutagens. Alcohol is an example of a chemical carcinogen that is not a mutagen. Such chemicals may promote cancers through stimulating the rate of cell division. Faster rates of replication leaves less time for repair enzymes to repair damaged DNA during DNA replication, increasing the likelihood of a mutation.

Decades of research has demonstrated the link between tobacco use and cancer in the lung, larynx, head, neck, stomach, bladder, kidney, oesophagus and pancreas. Tobacco smoke contains over fifty known carcinogens, including nitrosamines and polycyclic aromatic hydrocarbons. Tobacco is responsible for about one in three of all cancer deaths in the developed world, and about one in five worldwide. Indeed, lung cancer death rates in the United States have mirrored smoking patterns, with increases in smoking followed by dramatic increases in lung cancer death rates and, more recently, decreases in smoking followed by decreases in lung cancer death rates in men. However, the numbers of smokers worldwide is still rising, leading to what some organizations have described as the *tobacco epidemic.*

Ionizing Radiation

Sources of ionizing radiation, such as radon gas, can cause cancer. Prolonged exposure to ultraviolet radiation from the sun can lead to melanoma and other skin malignancies. It is estimated that 2% of future cancers will be due to current CT scans.

Non-ionizing radio frequency radiation from mobile phones and other similar RF sources has also been proposed as a cause of cancer, but there is currently little established evidence of such a link.

Infection

Some cancers can be caused by infection. This is especially true in animals such as birds, but also in humans, with viruses responsible for up to 20% of human cancers worldwide. These include human papillomavirus (cervical carcinoma), human polyomaviruses (mesothelioma, brain tumors), Epstein-Barr virus (B-cell lymphoproliferative disease and nasopharyngeal carcinoma), Kaposi's sarcoma herpesvirus (Kaposi's Sarcoma and primary effusion lymphomas), hepatitis B and hepatitis C viruses (hepatocellular carcinoma), Human T-cell leukemia virus-1 (T-cell leukemias), and Helicobacter pylori (gastric carcinoma).

Experimental and epidemiological data imply a causative role for viruses and they appear to be the second most important risk factor for cancer development in humans, exceeded only by tobacco usage. The mode of virally induced tumors can be divided into two, *acutely transforming* or *slowly transforming*. In acutely transforming viruses, the virus carries an overactive oncogene called viral-oncogene (v-onc), and the infected cell is transformed as soon as v-onc is expressed. In contrast, in slowly transforming viruses, the virus genome is inserts near a proto-oncogene in the host genome. The viral promoter or other transcription regulation elements then cause overexpression of that proto-oncogene. This induces uncontrolled cell division. Because the site of insertion is not specific to proto-oncogenes and the chance of insertion near any proto-oncogene is low, slowly transforming viruses will cause tumors much longer after infection than the acutely transforming viruses.

Hepatitis viruses, including hepatitis B and hepatitis C, can induce a chronic viral infection that leads to liver cancer in 0.47% of hepatitis B patients per year (especially in Asia, less so in North America), and in 1.4% of hepatitis C carriers per year. Liver cirrhosis, whether from chronic viral hepatitis infection or alcoholism, is associated with the development of liver cancer, and the combination of cirrhosis and viral hepatitis presents the highest risk of liver cancer development. Worldwide, liver cancer is one of the most common, and most deadly, cancers due to a huge burden of viral hepatitis transmission and disease.

Advances in cancer research have made a vaccine designed to prevent cancer available. In 2006, the U.S. Food and Drug Administration approved a human papilloma virus vaccine, called Gardasil. The vaccine protects against four HPV types, which together cause 70% of cervical cancers and 90% of genital warts. In March 2007, the US Centres for Disease Control and Prevention (CDC) Advisory Committee on Immunization Practices (ACIP) officially recommended that females aged 11–12 receive the vaccine, and indicated that females as young as age 9 and as old as age 26 are also candidates for immunization.

In addition to viruses, researchers have noted a connection between bacteria and certain cancers. The most prominent example is the link between chronic infection of the wall of the stomach with *Helicobacter pylori* and gastric cancer. Although only a minority of those infected with *Helicobacter* go on to develop cancer, since this pathogen is quite common it is probably responsible for most of these cancers.

Hormonal Imbalances

Some hormones can act in a similar manner to non-mutagenic carcinogens in that they may stimulate excessive cell growth.

Immune System Dysfunction

HIV is associated with a number of malignancies, including Kaposi's sarcoma, non-Hodgkin's lymphoma, and HPV-associated malignancies such as anal cancer and cervical cancer. AIDS-defining illnesses have long included these diagnoses. The increased incidence of malignancies in HIV patients points to the breakdown of immune surveillance as a possible etiology of cancer. Certain other immune deficiency states (e.g. common variable immunodeficiency and IgA deficiency) are also associated with increased risk of malignancy.

Heredity

Most forms of cancer are *sporadic*, meaning that there is no inherited cause of the cancer. There are, however, a number of recognised syndromes where there is an inherited predisposition to cancer, often due to a defect in a gene that protects against tumour formation. Famous examples are:

- certain inherited mutations in the genes *BRCA1* and *BRCA2* are associated with an elevated risk of breast cancer and ovarian cancer
- tumors of various endocrine organs in multiple endocrine neoplasia (MEN types 1, 2a, 2b)
- Li-Fraumeni syndrome (various tumors such as osteosarcoma, breast cancer, soft tissue sarcoma, brain tumors) due to mutations of p53
- Turcot syndrome (brain tumors and colonic polyposis)
- Familial adenomatous polyposis an inherited mutation of the *APC* gene that leads to early onset of colon carcinoma.
- Hereditary nonpolyposis colorectal cancer (HNPCC, also known as Lynch syndrome) can include familial cases of colon cancer, uterine cancer, gastric cancer, and ovarian cancer, without a preponderance of colon polyps.
- Retinoblastoma, when occurring in young children, is due to a hereditary mutation in the retinoblastoma gene.
- Down syndrome patients, who have an extra chromosome 21, are known to develop malignancies such as leukemia and testicular cancer, though the reasons for this difference are not well understood.

Other Causes

Excepting the rare transmissions that occur with pregnancies and only a marginal few organ donors, cancer is generally not a transmissible disease. The main reason for this is tissue graft rejection caused by MHC incompatibility. In humans and other vertebrates, the immune system uses MHC antigens to differentiate between "self" and "non-self" cells because these antigens are different from person to person. When non-self antigens are encountered, the immune system reacts against the appropriate cell. Such reactions may protect against tumour cell engraftment by eliminating implanted cells. In the United States, approximately 3,500 pregnant women have a malignancy annually, and transplacental transmission of acute leukaemia, lymphoma, melanoma and carcinoma from mother to fetus has been observed. The development of donor-derived tumors from organ transplants is exceedingly rare. The main cause of organ transplant associated tumors seems to be malignant melanoma, that was undetected at the time of organ harvest. though other cases exist In fact, cancer from one organism will usually grow in another organism of that species, as long as they share the same histocompatibility genes, proven using mice; however this would never happen in a real-world setting except as described above.

In non-humans, a few types of transmissible cancer have been described, wherein the cancer spreads between animals by transmission of the tumour cells themselves. This phenomenon is seen in dogs with Sticker's sarcoma, also known as canine transmissible venereal tumour, as well as Devil facial tumour disease in Tasmanian devils.

Pathophysiology

Cancer is fundamentally a disease of regulation of tissue growth. In order for a normal cell to transform into a cancer cell, genes which regulate cell growth and differentiation must be altered. Genetic changes can occur at many levels, from gain or loss of entire chromosomes to a mutation affecting a single DNA nucleotide. There are two broad categories of genes which are affected by these changes. Oncogenes may be normal genes which are expressed at inappropriately high levels, or altered genes which have novel properties. In either case, expression of these genes promotes the malignant phenotype of cancer cells. Tumour suppressor genes are genes which inhibit cell division, survival, or other properties of cancer cells. Tumour suppressor genes are often disabled by cancer-promoting genetic changes. Typically, changes in many genes are required to transform a normal cell into a cancer cell.

There is a diverse classification scheme for the various genomic changes which may contribute to the generation of cancer cells. Most of these changes are mutations, or changes in the nucleotide sequence of genomic DNA. Aneuploidy, the presence of an abnormal number of chromosomes, is one genomic change which is not a mutation, and may involve either gain or loss of one or more chromosomes through errors in mitosis.

Large-scale mutations involve the deletion or gain of a portion of a chromosome. Genomic amplification occurs when a cell gains many copies (often 20 or more) of a small chromosomal locus, usually containing one or more oncogenes and adjacent genetic material. Translocation occurs when two separate chromosomal regions become abnormally fused, often at a characteristic location. A well-known example of this is the Philadelphia chromosome, or translocation of chromosomes 9 and 22, which occurs in chronic myelogenous leukemia, and results in production of the BCR-abl fusion protein, an oncogenic tyrosine kinase.

Small-scale mutations include point mutations, deletions, and insertions, which may occur in the promoter of a gene and affect its expression, or may occur in the gene's coding sequence and alter the function or stability of its protein product. Disruption of a single gene may also result from integration of genomic material from a DNA virus or retrovirus, and such an event may also result in the expression of viral oncogenes in the affected cell and its descendants.

Prevention

Cancer prevention is defined as active measures to decrease the incidence of cancer. Greater than 30% of cancer is preventable via avoiding risk factors including: tobacco, overweight or obesity, low fruit and vegetable intake, physical inactivity, alcohol, sexually transmitted infection, air pollution. This can be accomplished by avoiding carcinogens or altering their metabolism, pursuing a lifestyle or diet that modifies cancer-causing factors and/or medical intervention (chemoprevention, treatment of pre-malignant lesions). The epidemiological concept of "prevention" is usually defined as either primary prevention, for people who have not been diagnosed with a particular disease, or secondary prevention, aimed at reducing recurrence or complications of a previously diagnosed illness.

But the EPIC study published in 2010, tracking the eating habits of 478,000 Europeans suggested that consuming lots of fruits and vegetables has little if any effect on preventing cancer.

Modifiable Factors

The vast majority of cancer risk factors are environmental or lifestyle-related, leading to the claim that cancer is a largely preventable disease. Examples of modifiable cancer risk factors include alcohol consumption (associated with increased risk of oral, esophageal, breast, and other cancers), smoking (80% of women with lung cancer have smoked in the past, and 90% of men), physical inactivity (associated with increased risk of colon, breast, and possibly other cancers), and being overweight/obese (associated with colon, breast, endometrial, and possibly other cancers). Based on epidemiologic evidence, it is now thought that avoiding excessive alcohol consumption may contribute to reductions in risk of certain cancers; however, compared with tobacco exposure, the magnitude of effect is modest or small and the strength of evidence is often weaker. Other lifestyle and environmental factors known to affect cancer risk (either beneficially or detrimentally) include certain sexually transmitted diseases (such as those conveyed by the human papillomavirus), the use of exogenous hormones, exposure to ionizing radiation and ultraviolet radiation from the sun or from tanning beds, and certain occupational and chemical exposures.

Every year, at least 200,000 people die worldwide from cancer related to their workplace. Millions of workers run the risk of developing cancers such as lung cancer and mesothelioma from inhaling asbestos fibres and tobacco smoke, or leukemia from exposure to benzene at their workplaces. Currently, most cancer deaths caused by occupational risk factors occur in the developed world. It is estimated that approximately 20,000 cancer deaths and 40,000 new cases of cancer each year in the U.S. are attributable to occupation.

Diet

The consensus on diet and cancer is that obesity increases the risk of developing cancer. Particular dietary practices often explain differences in cancer incidence in different countries (e.g. gastric cancer is more common in Japan, while colon cancer is more common in the United States. In this example the preceding consideration of Haplogroups are excluded). Studies have shown that immigrants develop the risk of their new country, often within one generation, suggesting a substantial link between diet and cancer. Whether reducing obesity in a population also reduces cancer incidence is unknown.

Despite frequent reports of particular substances (including foods) having a beneficial or detrimental effect on cancer risk, few of these have an established link to cancer. These reports are often based on studies in cultured cell media or animals. Public health recommendations cannot be made based on these studies until they have been validated in an observational (or occasionally a prospective interventional) trial in humans.

Proposed dietary interventions for primary cancer risk reduction generally gain support from epidemiological association studies. Examples of such studies include reports that reduced meat consumption is associated with decreased risk of colon cancer, and reports that consumption of coffee is associated with a reduced risk of liver cancer. Studies have linked consumption of grilled meat to an increased risk of stomach cancer, colon cancer, breast cancer, and pancreatic cancer, a phenomenon which could be due to the presence of carcinogens such as benzopyrene in foods cooked at high temperatures. A 2005 secondary prevention study showed that consumption of a plant-based diet and lifestyle changes resulted in a reduction in cancer markers in a group of men with prostate cancer who were using no conventional treatments at the time. These results were amplified by a 2006 study. Over 2,400 women were studied, half randomly assigned to a normal diet, the other half assigned to a diet containing less than 20% calories from fat. The women on the low fat diet were found to have a markedly lower risk of breast cancer recurrence, in the interim report of December, 2006.

Recent studies have also demonstrated potential links between some forms of cancer and high consumption of refined sugars and other simple carbohydrates. Although the degree of correlation and the degree of causality is still debated, some organizations have in fact begun to recommend reducing intake of refined sugars and starches as part of their cancer prevention regimens.

In November 2007, the American Institute for Cancer Research (AICR), in conjunction with the World Cancer Research Fund (WCRF), published *Food, Nutrition, Physical Activity and the Prevention of Cancer: a Global Perspective*, "the most current and comprehensive analysis of the literature on diet, physical activity and cancer". The WCRF/AICR Expert Report lists 10 recommendations that people can follow to help reduce their risk of developing cancer, including the following dietary guidelines: (1) reducing intake of foods and drinks that promote weight gain, namely energy-dense foods and sugary drinks, (2) eating mostly foods of plant origin, (3) limiting intake of red meat and avoiding processed meat, (4) limiting consumption of alcoholic beverages, and (5) reducing intake of salt and avoiding mouldy cereals (grains) or pulses (legumes).

Some mushrooms offer an anti-cancer effect, which is thought to be linked to their ability to up-regulate the immune system. Some mushrooms known for this effect include, Reishi, *Agaricus blazei*, Maitake, and *Trametes versicolor*. Research suggests the compounds in medicinal mushrooms most responsible for up-regulating the immune system and providing an anti-cancer effect, are a diverse collection of polysaccharide compounds, particularly beta-glucans. Beta-glucans are known as "biological response modifiers", and their ability to activate the immune system is well documented. Specifically, beta-glucans stimulate the innate branch of the immune system. Research has shown beta-glucans have the ability to stimulate macrophage, NK cells, T cells, and immune system cytokines. The mechanisms in which beta-glucans stimulate the immune system is only partially understood. One mechanism in which beta-glucans are able to activate the immune system, is by interacting with the Macrophage-1 antigen (CD18) receptor on immune cells.

Vitamins

Vitamin supplementation has not been proven effective in the prevention of cancer. The components of food are also proving to be more numerous and varied than previously understood, so patients are increasingly advised to consume fruits and vegetables for maximal health benefits.

Vitamin D

Low levels of vitamin D is correlated with increased cancer risk. Whether this relationship is causal is yet to be determined.

Beta Carotene

Beta-carotene supplementation has been found to increase slightly, but not significantly risks of lung cancer.

Folic Acid

Folic acid supplementation has not been found effective in preventing colon cancer and may increase colon polyps.

Chemoprevention

The concept that medications could be used to prevent cancer is an attractive one, and many high-quality clinical trials support the use of such chemoprevention in defined circumstances.

Daily use of tamoxifen, a selective estrogen receptor modulator (SERM), typically for 5 years, has been demonstrated to reduce the risk of developing breast cancer in high-risk women by about 50%.

A recent study reported that the selective estrogen receptor modulator raloxifene has similar benefits to tamoxifen in preventing breast cancer in high-risk women, with a more favourable side effect profile.

Raloxifene is a SERM like tamoxifen; it has been shown (in the STAR trial) to reduce the risk of breast cancer in high-risk women equally as well as tamoxifen. In this trial, which studied almost 20,000 women, raloxifene had fewer side effects than tamoxifen, though it did permit more DCIS to form.

Finasteride, a 5-alpha-reductase inhibitor, has been shown to lower the risk of prostate cancer, though it seems to mostly prevent low-grade tumors. The effect of COX-2 inhibitors such as rofecoxib and celecoxib upon the risk of colon polyps have been studied in familial adenomatous polyposis patients and in the general population. In both groups, there were significant reductions in colon polyp incidence, but this came at the price of increased cardiovascular toxicity.

Genetic Testing

Genetic testing for high-risk individuals is already available for certain cancer-related genetic mutations. Carriers of genetic mutations that increase risk for cancer incidence can undergo enhanced surveillance, chemoprevention, or risk-reducing surgery. Early identification of inherited genetic risk for cancer, along with cancer-preventing interventions such as surgery or enhanced surveillance, can be lifesaving for high-risk individuals.

Vaccination

Prophylactic vaccines have been developed to prevent infection by oncogenic infectious agents such as viruses, and therapeutic vaccines are in development to stimulate an immune response against cancer-specific epitopes.

As reported above, a preventive human papillomavirus vaccine exists that targets certain sexually transmitted strains of human papillomavirus that are associated with the development of cervical cancer and genital warts. The only two HPV vaccines on the market as of October 2007 are Gardasil and Cervarix. There is also a hepatitis B vaccine, which prevents infection with the hepatitis B virus, an infectious agent that can cause liver cancer. A canine melanoma vaccine has also been developed.

Screening

Cancer screening is an attempt to detect unsuspected cancers in an asymptomatic population. Screening tests suitable for large numbers of healthy people must be relatively affordable, safe, noninvasive procedures with acceptably low rates of false positive results. If signs of cancer are detected, more definitive and invasive follow up tests are performed to confirm the diagnosis.

Screening for cancer can lead to earlier diagnosis in specific cases. Early diagnosis may lead to extended life, but may also falsely prolong the lead time to death through lead time bias or length time bias.

A number of different screening tests have been developed for different malignancies. Breast cancer screening can be done by breast self-examination, though this approach was discredited by a 2005 study in over 300,000 Chinese women. Screening for breast cancer with mammograms has been shown to reduce the average stage of diagnosis of breast cancer in a population. Stage of diagnosis in a country has been shown to decrease within ten years of introduction of mammographic screening programs. Colorectal cancer can be detected through fecal occult blood testing and colonoscopy, which reduces both colon cancer incidence and mortality, presumably through the detection and removal of pre-malignant polyps. Similarly, cervical cytology testing (using the Pap smear) leads to the identification and excision of precancerous lesions. Over time, such testing has been followed by a dramatic reduction of cervical cancer incidence and mortality. Testicular self-examination is recommended for men beginning at the age of 15 years to detect testicular cancer. Prostate cancer can be screened using a digital rectal exam along with prostate specific antigen (PSA) blood testing, though some authorities (such as the US Preventive Services Task Force) recommend against routinely screening all men.

Screening for cancer is controversial in cases when it is not yet known if the test actually saves lives. The controversy arises when it is not clear if the benefits of screening outweigh the risks of follow-up diagnostic tests and cancer treatments. For example: when screening for prostate cancer, the PSA test may detect small cancers that would never become life threatening, but once detected will lead to treatment. This situation, called overdiagnosis, puts men at risk for complications from unnecessary treatment such as surgery or radiation. Follow up procedures used to diagnose prostate cancer (prostate biopsy) may cause side effects, including bleeding and infection. Prostate cancer treatment may cause incontinence (inability to control urine flow) and erectile dysfunction (erections inadequate for intercourse). Similarly, for breast cancer, there have recently been criticisms that breast screening programs in some countries cause more problems than they solve. This is because screening of women in the general population will result in a large number of women with false positive results which require extensive follow-up investigations to exclude cancer, leading to having a high number-to-treat (or number-to-screen) to prevent or catch a single case of breast cancer early.

Cervical cancer screening via the Pap smear has the best cost-benefit profile of all the forms of cancer screening from a public health perspective as, largely caused by a virus, it has clear risk factors (sexual contact), and the natural progression of cervical cancer is that it normally spreads slowly over a number of years therefore giving more time for the screening program to catch it early. Moreover, the test is easy to perform and relatively cheap.

For these reasons, it is important that the benefits and risks of diagnostic procedures and treatment be taken into account when considering whether to undertake cancer screening. Use of medical imaging to search for cancer in people without clear symptoms is similarly marred with problems. There is a significant risk of detection of what has been recently called an *incidentaloma* - a benign lesion that may be interpreted as a malignancy and be subjected to potentially dangerous investigations. Recent studies of CT scan-based screening for lung cancer in smokers have had equivocal results, and systematic screening is not recommended as of July 2007. Randomized clinical trials of plain-film chest X-rays to screen for lung cancer in smokers have shown no benefit for this approach. Canine cancer detection has shown promise, but is still in the early stages of research.

Diagnosis

Most cancers are initially recognized either because signs or symptoms appear or through screening. Neither of these lead to a definitive diagnosis, which usually requires the opinion of a pathologist, a type of physician (medical doctor) who specializes in the diagnosis of cancer and other diseases. People with suspected cancer are investigated with medical tests. These commonly include blood tests, X-rays, CT scans and endoscopy.

Pathology

A cancer may be suspected for a variety of reasons, but the definitive diagnosis of most malignancies must be confirmed by histological examination of the cancerous cells by a pathologist. Tissue can be obtained from a biopsy or surgery. Many biopsies (such as those of the skin, breast or liver) can be done in a doctor's office. Biopsies of other organs are performed under anesthesia and require surgery in an operating room.

The tissue diagnosis given by the pathologist indicates the type of cell that is proliferating, its histological grade, genetic abnormalities, and other features of the tumour. Together, this information is useful to evaluate the prognosis of the patient and to choose the best treatment. Cytogenetics and immunohistochemistry are other types of testing that the pathologist may perform on the tissue specimen. These tests may provide information about the molecular changes (such as mutations, fusion genes, and numerical chromosome changes) that has happened in the cancer cells, and may thus also indicate the future behavior of the cancer (prognosis) and best treatment.

Management

Many management options for cancer exist including: chemotherapy, radiation therapy, surgery, immunotherapy, monoclonal antibody therapy and other methods. Which are used depends upon the location and grade of the tumour and the stage of the disease, as well as the general state of a person's health. Experimental cancer treatments are also under development.

Complete removal of the cancer without damage to the rest of the body is the goal of treatment. Sometimes this can be accomplished by surgery, but the propensity of cancers to invade adjacent tissue or to spread to distant sites by microscopic metastasis often limits its effectiveness. Surgery often required the removal of a wide surgical margin or a free margin. The width of the free margin depends on the type of the cancer, the method of removal (CCPDMA, Mohs surgery, POMA, etc.). The margin can be as little as 1 mm for basal cell cancer using CCPDMA or Mohs surgery, to several centimeters for aggressive cancers. The effectiveness of chemotherapy is often limited by toxicity to other tissues in the body. Radiation can also cause damage to normal tissue. Because "cancer" refers to a class of diseases, it is unlikely that there will ever be a single "cure for cancer" any more than there will be a single treatment for all infectious diseases. Angiogenesis inhibitors were once thought to have potential as a "silver bullet" treatment applicable to many types of cancer, but this has not been the case in practice.

Prognosis

Cancer has a reputation as a deadly disease. While this certainly applies to certain particular types, the truths behind the historical connotations of cancer are increasingly overturned by advances in medical care. Some types of cancer have a prognosis that is substantially better than nonmalignant diseases such as heart failure and stroke.

Progressive and disseminated malignant disease has a substantial impact on a cancer patient's quality of life, and many cancer treatments (such as chemotherapy) may have severe side-effects. In the advanced stages of cancer, many patients need extensive care, affecting family members and friends. Palliative care solutions may include permanent or "respite" hospice nursing.

Epidemiology

As of 2004, worldwide cancer caused 13% of all deaths (7.4 million). The leading causes were: lung cancer (1.3 million deaths/year), stomach cancer (803,000 deaths), colorectal cancer (639,000 deaths), liver cancer (610,000 deaths), and breast cancer (519,000 deaths). Greater than 30% of cancer is preventable via avoiding risk factors including: tobacco, overweight or obesity, low fruit and vegetable intake, physical inactivity, alcohol, sexually transmitted infections, and air pollution.

In the United States, cancer is responsible for 25% of all deaths with 30% of these from lung cancer. The most commonly occurring cancer in men is prostate cancer (about 25% of new cases) and in women is breast cancer (also about 25%). Cancer can occur in children and adolescents, but it is uncommon (about 150 cases per million in the U.S.), with leukemia the most common. In the first year of life the incidence is about 230 cases per million in the U.S., with the most common being neuroblastoma.

In the developed world, one in three people will develop cancer during their lifetimes. If *all* cancer patients survived and cancer occurred *randomly*, the lifetime odds of developing an second primary cancer would be one in nine. However, cancer survivors have an increased risk of developing a second primary cancer, and the odds are about two in nine. About half of these second primaries can be attributed to the normal one-in-nine risk associated with random chance. The increased risk is believed to be primarily due to the same risk factors that produced the first cancer, such as the person's genetic profile, alcohol and tobacco use, obesity, and environmental exposures, and partly due, to the treatment for the first cancer, which typically includes mutagenic chemotherapeutic drugs or radiation. Cancer survivors may also be more likely to comply with recommended screening, and thus may be more likely than average to detect cancers.

History

Today, the Greek term carcinoma is the medical term for a malignant tumour derived from epithelial cells. It is Celsus who translated *carcinos* into the Latin *cancer*, also meaning crab. Galen used "*oncos*" to describe *all* tumours, the root for the modern word oncology. Hippocrates described several kinds of cancers. He called benign tumours *oncos*, Greek for swelling, and malignant tumours *carcinos*, Greek for crab or crayfish. This name comes from the appearance of the cut surface of a solid malignant tumour, with "the veins stretched on all sides as the animal the crab has its feet, whence it derives its name". He later added the suffix *-oma*, Greek for swelling, giving the name *carcinoma*. Since it was against Greek tradition to open the body, Hippocrates only described and made drawings of outwardly visible tumors on the skin, nose, and breasts. Treatment was based on the humor theory of four bodily fluids (black and yellow bile, blood, and phlegm). According to the patient's humor, treatment consisted of diet, blood-letting, and/or laxatives. Through the centuries it was discovered that cancer could occur anywhere in the body, but humor-theory based treatment remained popular until the 19th century with the discovery of cells. The oldest known description and surgical treatment of cancer was discovered in Egypt and dates back to approximately 1600 B.C. The Papyrus describes 8 cases of ulcers of the breast that were treated by cauterization, with a tool called "the fire drill." The writing says about the disease, "There is no treatment."

Another very early surgical treatment for cancer was described in the 1020s by Avicenna (Ibn Sina) in *The Canon of Medicine*. He stated that the excision should be radical and that all diseased tissue should be removed, which included the use of amputation or the removal of veins running in the direction of the tumour. He also recommended the use of cauterization for the area treated if necessary.

In the 16th and 17th centuries, it became more acceptable for doctors to dissect bodies to discover the cause of death. The German professor Wilhelm Fabry believed that breast cancer was caused by a milk clot in a mammary duct. The Dutch professor Francois de la Boe Sylvius, a follower of Descartes, believed that all disease was the outcome of chemical processes, and that acidic lymph fluid was the cause of cancer. His contemporary Nicolaes Tulp believed that cancer was a poison that slowly spreads, and concluded that it was contagious.

The first cause of cancer was identified by British surgeon Percivall Pott, who discovered in 1775 that cancer of the scrotum was a common disease among chimney sweeps. The work of other individual physicians led to various insights, but when physicians started working together they could make firmer conclusions. With the widespread use of the microscope in the 18th century, it was discovered that the 'cancer poison' spread from the primary tumour through the lymph nodes to other sites ("metastasis"). This view of the disease was first formulated by the English surgeon Campbell De Morgan between 1871 and 1874. The use of surgery to treat cancer had poor results due to problems with hygiene. The renowned Scottish surgeon Alexander Monro saw only 2 breast tumour patients out of 60 surviving surgery for two years. In the 19th century, asepsis improved surgical hygiene and as the survival statistics went up, surgical removal of the tumour became the primary treatment for cancer. With the exception of William Coley who in the late 1800s felt that the rate of cure after surgery had been higher *before* asepsis (and who injected bacteria into tumors with mixed results), cancer treatment became dependent on the individual art of the surgeon at removing a tumour. During the same period, the idea that the body was made up of various tissues, that in turn were made up of millions of cells, laid rest the humor-theories about chemical imbalances in the body. The age of cellular pathology was born. The genetic basis of cancer was recognised in 1902 by the German zoologist Theodor Boveri, professor of zoology at Munich and later in Würzburg. He discovered a method to generate cells with multiple copies of the centrosome, a structure he discovered and named. He postulated that chromosomes were distinct and transmitted different inheritance factors. He suggested that mutations of the chromosomes could generate a cell with unlimited growth potential which could be passed onto its descendants. He proposed the existence of cell cycle check points, tumour suppressor genes and oncogenes. He speculated that cancers might be caused or promoted by radiation, physical or chemical insults or by pathogenic microorganisms.

When Marie Curie and Pierre Curie discovered radiation at the end of the 19th century, they stumbled upon the first effective non-surgical cancer treatment. With radiation also came the first signs of multi-disciplinary approaches to cancer treatment. The surgeon was no longer operating in isolation, but worked together with hospital radiologists to help patients. The complications in communication this brought, along with the necessity of the patient's treatment in a hospital facility rather than at home, also created a parallel process of compiling patient data into hospital files, which in turn led to the first statistical patient studies.

A founding paper of cancer epidemiology was the work of Janet Lane-Claypon, who published a comparative study in 1926 of 500 breast cancer cases and 500 control patients of the same background and lifestyle for the British Ministry of Health. Her ground-breaking work on cancer epidemiology was carried on by Richard Doll and

Austin Bradford Hill, who published "Lung Cancer and Other Causes of Death In Relation to Smoking. A Second Report on the Mortality of British Doctors" followed in 1956 (otherwise known as the British doctors study). Richard Doll left the London Medical Research Centre (MRC), to start the Oxford unit for Cancer epidemiology in 1968. With the use of computers, the unit was the first to compile large amounts of cancer data. Modern epidemiological methods are closely linked to current concepts of disease and public health policy. Over the past 50 years, great efforts have been spent on gathering data across medical practise, hospital, provincial, state, and even country boundaries to study the interdependence of environmental and cultural factors on cancer incidence. Cancer patient treatment and studies were restricted to individual physicians' practices until World War II, when medical research centres discovered that there were large international differences in disease incidence. This insight drove national public health bodies to make it possible to compile health data across practises and hospitals, a process that many countries do today. The Japanese medical community observed that the bone marrow of victims of the atomic bombings of Hiroshima and Nagasaki was completely destroyed. They concluded that diseased bone marrow could also be destroyed with radiation, and this led to the discovery of bone marrow transplants for leukemia. Since World War II, trends in cancer treatment are to improve on a micro-level the existing treatment methods, standardize them, and globalize them to find cures through epidemiology and international partnerships.

Research

Cancer research is the intense scientific effort to understand disease processes and discover possible therapies. The improved understanding of molecular biology and cellular biology due to cancer research has led to a number of new, effective treatments for cancer since President Nixon declared "War on Cancer" in 1971. Since 1971 the United States has invested over $200 billion on cancer research; that total includes money invested by public and private sectors and foundations. Despite this substantial investment, the country has seen a five percent decrease in the cancer death rate (adjusting for size and age of the population) between 1950 and 2005. Leading cancer research organizations and projects include the American Association for Cancer Research, the American Cancer Society (ACS), the American Society of Clinical Oncology, the European Organisation for Research and Treatment of Cancer, the National Cancer Institute, the National Comprehensive Cancer Network, and The Cancer Genome Atlas project at the NCI.

Chapter 4

Genetic Engineering

Genetic engineering, also called genetic modification, is the direct human manipulation of an organism's genetic material in a way that does not occur under natural conditions. It involves the use of recombinant DNA techniques, but does not include traditional animal and plant breeding or mutagenesis. Any organism that is generated using these techniques is considered to be a genetically modified organism. The first organisms genetically engineered were bacteria in 1973 and then mice in 1974. Insulin producing bacteria were commercialized in 1982 and genetically modified food has been sold since 1994.

The most common form of genetic engineering involves the insertion of new genetic material at an unspecified location in the host genome. This is accomplished by isolating and copying the genetic material of interest, generating a construct containing all the genetic elements for correct expression, and then inserting this construct into the host organism. Other forms of genetic engineering include gene targeting and knocking out specific genes via engineered nucleases such as zinc finger nucleases or engineered homing endonucleases.

Genetic engineering techniques have been applied in numerous fields including research, biotechnology, and medicine. Medicines such as insulin and human growth hormone are now produced in bacteria, experimental mice such as the oncomouse and the knockout mouse are being used for research purposes and insect resistant and/or herbicide tolerant crops have been commercialized. Genetically engineered plants and animals capable of producing biotechnology drugs more cheaply than current methods (called pharming) are also being developed and in 2009 the FDA approved the sale of the pharmaceutical protein antithrombin produced in the milk of genetically engineered goats.

Definition

Genetic engineering alters the genetic makeup of an organism using techniques that introduce heritable material prepared outside the organism either directly into the host or into a cell that is then fused or hybridized with the host. This involves using recombinant nucleic acid (DNA or RNA) techniques to form new combinations of heritable genetic material followed by the incorporation of that material either indirectly through a vector system or directly through micro-injection, macro-injection and micro-encapsulation techniques. Genetic engineering does not include traditional animal and plant breeding, in vitro fertilisation, induction of polyploidy, mutagenesis and cell fusion techniques that do not use recombinant nucleic acids or a genetically modified organism in the process. Cloning and stem cell research, although not considered genetic engineering, are closely related and genetic engineering can be used within them. Synthetic biology is an emerging discipline that takes genetic engineering a step further by introducing artificially synthesized genetic material from raw materials into an organism.

If genetic material from another species is added to the host, the resulting organism is called transgenic. If genetic material from the same species or a species that can naturally breed with the host is used the resulting organism is called cisgenic. Genetic engineering can also be used to remove genetic material from the target organism, creating a knock out organism. In Europe genetic modification is synonymous with genetic engineering while within the United States of America it can also refer to conventional breeding methods.

History

Humans have altered the genomes of species for thousands of years through artificial selection and more recently mutagenesis. Genetic engineering as the direct manipulation of DNA by humans outside breeding and mutations has only existed since the 1970s. The term "genetic engineering" was first coined by Jack Williamson in his science fiction novel *Dragon's Island*, published in 1951, one year before DNA's role in heredity was confirmed by Alfred Hershey and Martha Chase, and two years before James Watson and Francis Crick showed that the DNA molecule has a double-helix structure.

In 1972 Paul Berg created the first recombinant DNA molecules by combined DNA from the monkey virus SV40 with that of the lambda virus. In 1973 Herbert Boyer and Stanley Cohen created the first transgenic organism by inserting antibiotic resistance genes into the plasmid of an *E. coli* bacterium. A year later Rudolf Jaenisch created a transgenic mouse by introducing foreign DNA into its embryo, making it the world's first transgenic animal. In 1976 Genentech, the first genetic engineering company was founded by Herbert Boyer and Robert Swanson and a year later and the company produced a human protein (somatostatin) in *E.coli*. Genentech announced the production of genetically engineered human insulin in 1978. In 1980, the U.S. Supreme Court in the Diamond v. Chakrabarty case ruled that genetically altered life could be patented. The insulin produced by bacteria, branded humulin, was approved for release by the Food and Drug Administration in 1982.

The first field trials of genetically engineered plants occurred in France and the USA in 1986, tobacco plants were engineered to be resistant to herbicides. The People's Republic of China was the first country to commercialize transgenic plants, introducing a virus-resistant tobacco in 1992.

In 1994 Calgene attained approval to commercially release the Flavr Savr tomato, a tomato engineered to have a longer shelf life. In 1994, the European Union approved tobacco engineered to be resistant to the herbicide bromoxynil, making it the first genetically engineered crop commercialized in Europe.

In 1995, Bt Potato was approved safe by the Environmental Protection Agency, making it the first pesticide producing crop to be approved in the USA. In 2009 11 transgenic crops were grown commercially in 25 countries, the largest of which by area grown were the USA, Brazil, Argentina, India, Canada, China, Paraguay and South Africa.

In 2010, scientists at the J. Craig Venter Institute, announced that they had created the first synthetic bacterial genome, and added it to a cell containing no DNA. The resulting bacterium, named Synthia, was the world's first synthetic life form.

Process

Isolating the Gene

First, the gene to be inserted into the genetically modified organism must be chosen and isolated. Presently, most genes transferred into plants provide protection against insects or tolerance to herbicides. In animals the majority of genes used are growth hormone genes. Once chosen the genes must be isolated. This typically involves multiplying the gene using polymerase chain reaction (PCR). If the chosen gene or the donor organism's genome has been well studied it may be present in a genetic library. If the DNA sequence is known, but no copies of the gene are available, it can be artificially synthesized. Once isolated, the gene is inserted into a bacterial plasmid.

Constructs

The gene to be inserted into the genetically modified organism must be combined with other genetic elements in order for it to work properly. The gene can also be modified at this stage for better expression or effectiveness. As well as the gene to be inserted most constructs contain a promoter and terminator region as well as a selectable marker gene.

The promoter region initiates transcription of the gene and can be used to control the location and level of gene expression, while the terminator region ends transcription. The selectable marker, which in most cases confers antibiotic resistance to the organism it is expressed in, is needed to determine which cells are transformed with the new gene. The constructs are made using recombinant DNA techniques, such as restriction digests, ligations and molecular cloning.

Gene Targeting

Gene targeting (also, replacement strategy based on homologous recombination) is a genetic technique that uses homologous recombination to change an endogenous gene. The method can be used to delete a gene, remove exons, add a gene, and introduce point mutations. Gene targeting can be permanent or conditional. Conditions can be a specific time during development / life of the organism or limitation to a specific tissue, for example. Gene targeting requires the creation of a specific vector for each gene of interest. However, it can be used for any gene, regardless of transcriptional activity or gene size.

Methods

Gene targeting methods are established for several model organisms and may vary depending on the species used. In general, a targeting construct made out of DNA is generated in bacteria. It typically contains part of the gene to be targeted, a reporter gene, and a (dominant) selectable marker.

To target genes in mice, this construct is then inserted into mouse embryonic stem cells in culture. After cells with the correct insertion have been selected, they can be used to contribute to a mouse's tissue via embryo injection. Finally, chimeric mice where the modified cells made up the reproductive organs are selected for via breeding. After this step the entire body of the mouse is based on the previously selected embryonic stem cell.

To target genes in moss, this construct is incubated together with freshly isolated protoplasts and with Polyethylene glycol. As mosses are haploid organisms, regenerating moss filaments (protonema) can directly be screened for gene targeting, either by treatment with antibiotics or with PCR. Unique among plants, this procedure for reverse genetics is as efficient as in yeast. Using modified procedures, gene targeting has also been successfully applied to cattle, sheep, swine, and many fungi.

Comparison with Gene Trapping

Gene trapping is based on random insertion of a cassette while gene targeting targets a specific gene. Cassettes can be used for many different things while the flanking homology regions of gene targeting cassettes need to be adapted for each gene. This makes gene trapping more easily amenable for large scale projects than targeting. On the other hand, gene targeting can be used for genes with low transcriptions that would go undetected in a trap screen. Also, the probability of trapping increases with intron size. For gene targeting these compact genes are just as easily altered.

Applications

Gene targeting has been widely used to study human genetic diseases by removing "knock-out", or adding "knock-in", specific mutations of interest to a variety of models. Previously used to engineer rat cell models, advances in gene targeting technologies are enabling the creation of a new wave of isogenic human disease models. These models are the most accurate in-vitro models available to researchers to date, and are facilitating the development of new personalised drugs and diagnostics, particularly in the field of cancer.

2007 Nobel Prize

Mario R. Capecchi, Martin J. Evans and Oliver Smithies were declared laureates of the 2007 Nobel Prize in Physiology or Medicine for their work on "principles for introducing specific gene modifications in mice by the use of embryonic stem cells", or gene targeting.

Transformation (Genetics)

In molecular biology transformation is the genetic alteration of a cell resulting from the direct uptake, incorporation and expression of exogenous genetic material (exogenous DNA) from its surrounding and taken up through the cell membrane(s). Transformation occurs most commonly in bacteria and in some species occurs naturally. Transformation can also be effected by artificial means. Bacteria that are capable of being transformed, whether naturally or artificially, are called competent. Transformation is one of three processes by which a exogenous genetic material may be introduced into bacterial cell, the other two being conjugation (transfer of genetic material between two bacterial cells in direct contact), and transduction (injection of foreign DNA by a bacteriophage into the host). Transformation may also used to describe the insertion of new genetic material into nonbacterial cells including animal and plant cells, however, because transformation has a special meaning in relation to animal cells indicating progression to a cancerous state, the term should be avoided for animal cells when describing introduction of exogenous genetic material. Introduction of foreign DNA into eukaryotic cells is usually called "transfection".

History

Transformation was first demonstrated in 1928 by Frederick Griffith, an English bacteriologist searching for a vaccine against bacterial pneumonia. Griffith discovered that a harmless strain of *Streptococcus pneumoniae* could be made virulent after being exposed to heat-killed virulent strains. Griffith hypothesized that some "transforming factor" from the heat-killed strain was responsible for making the harmless strain virulent. In 1944 this "transforming factor" was identified as being genetic by Oswald Avery, Colin MacLeod, and Maclyn McCarty. They isolated DNA from a virulent strain of *S. pneumoniae* and using just this DNA were able to make a harmless strain virulent. They called this uptake and incorporation of DNA by bacteria "transformation."

The results of Avery et al.'s experiments were at first sceptically received by the scientific community and it was not until the development of genetic markers and the discovery of other methods of genetic transfer (conjugation in 1947 and transduction in 1953) by Joshua Lederberg that Avery's experiments were accepted. Transformation did not become routine procedure in laboratories until 1972 when Stanley Cohen, Annie Chang and Leslie Hsu successfully transformed *Escherichia coli* by treating the bacteria with calcium chloride. This created an efficient and convenient procedure for transforming bacteria and opened the way for molecular cloning in biotechnology and research.

Transformation using electroporation was developed in the late 1980s thus increasing the efficiency and number of bacterial strains that could be transformed. Transformation of animal and plant cells was also investigated with the first transgenic mouse being created by injecting a gene for a rat growth hormone into a mouse embryo in 1982. In 1907 a bacterium that caused plant tumours, *Agrobacterium tumefaciens*, was discovered and in the early 1970s the tumour inducing agent was found to be a DNA plasmid called the Ti plasmid. By removing the genes in the plasmid that caused the cancer and adding in novel genes researchers were able to infect plants with *A. tumefaciens* and let the bacteria insert their chosen DNA into the genomes of the plants. Not all plant cells are susceptible to infection by *A. tumefaciens* so other methods were developed including electroporation and micro-injection. Particle bombardment was made possible with the invention of the Biolistic Particle Delivery System (gene gun) by John Sanford in 1990.

Mechanisms

Bacteria

Bacteria transformation may be referred to as a stable genetic change brought about by the uptake of naked DNA (DNA without associated cells or proteins) and competence refers to the state of being able to take up exogenous DNA from the environment. Two forms of competence exist: natural and artificial.

Natural Competence

About 1% of bacterial species are capable of naturally taking up DNA under laboratory conditions; many more are able to take it up in their natural environments. Such bacteria carry sets of genes that provide the protein machinery to bring DNA across the cell membrane(s).

DNA material can be transferred between different strains of bacteria, in a process called horizontal gene transfer.

Artificial Competence

Artificial competence is induced by laboratory procedures and involves making the cell passively permeable to DNA by exposing it to conditions that do not normally occur in nature. Calcium chloride transformation is a method of promoting competence. Chilling cells in the presence of divalent cations such as Ca^{2+} (in $CaCl_2$) prepares the cell membrane to become permeable to plasmid DNA. The cells are incubated on ice with the DNA and then briefly heat shocked (e.g.,

42°C for 30–120 seconds) thus allowing the DNA to enter the cells. This method works very well for circular plasmid DNA. An excellent preparation of competent cells will give ~10^8 colonies per microgram of plasmid. A poor preparation will be about 10^4/mg or less. Good, non-commercial preparations should give 10^5 to 10^6 transformants per microgram of plasmid. The method, however, usually does not work well for linear DNA, such as fragments of chromosomal DNA, probably because the cell's native exonuclease enzymes rapidly degrade linear DNA. Interestingly, cells that are naturally competent are usually transformed more efficiently with linear DNA than with plasmid DNA.

Electroporation is another method of promoting competence. In the method the cells are briefly shocked with an electric field of 10-20 kV/cm that creates holes in the cell membrane through which the plasmid DNA enters. This method is amenable to the uptake of large plasmid DNA. After the electric shock the holes are rapidly closed by the cell's membrane-repair mechanisms.

The efficiency with which a competent culture can take up exogenous DNA and express its genes is known as Transformation efficiency.

Plasmid Transformation

In order to be stably maintained in the cell a plasmid DNA molecule must contain an origin of replication, which allows it to be replicated in the cell independent of the replication of the cell's own chromosome. Because transformation usually produces a mixture of relatively few transformed cells and an abundance of non-transformed cells a method is needed to identify the cells that have acquired the plasmid. The method usually consists of using a plasmid that contains a gene that gives the bacterial cells resistance to an antibiotic that they are naturally sensitive to. The mixture of cells are then plated on media that contains the antibiotic thus only the transformed cells are able to grow. Cells that did not take up the plasmid are killed in the media.

Another selection method called blue-white screen uses a plasmid that contains an antibiotic resistance gene and the lacZ gene. The lacZ gene codes for the lacZ-a subunit of the enzyme b-galactosidase, a homo-tetramer with each monomer composed of one lacZ-a subunit and one lacZ-w subunit. The method also requires an E. coli strain that possesses in its genome the code for only the lacZ-w subunit and not the lacZ-a subunit. One of the first steps in any transformation is the production of a recombined plasmid obtained by the successful ligation of the gene of interest into its corresponding vector, which in this method results in the disruption of lacZ because the gene of interest is inserted within the lacZ code. A cell that takes up a recombined plasmid would thus not be able to express the lacZ-a subunit and would, in turn, not be able to produce a functional b-galactosidase. Conversely, a cell that has taken up non-recombined plasmid (perhaps one formed by the ligation of the vector's own two ends) will express the lacZ-a subunit and thus produce a functional b-galactosidase. A cell that does not take up any plasmid is not conferred with antibiotic resistance and will die upon plating. Consequently, the blue-white screen method allows for the ready detection of not just transformed cells, but, most importantly, cells that have been transformed by a successfully recombined plasmid. Selection occurs as a result of the action of b-galactosidase on its substrate X-gal, which is included in the media along with the appropriate antibiotic. X-gal is a colorless, modified galactose sugar whose hydrolysis by b-galactosidase produces galactose and the pre-chromophore 5-bromo-4-chloro-3-hydroxyindole. The latter is subsequently oxidized to 5,5'-dibromo-4,4'-dichloro-indigo, an insoluble, blue product that is readily seen by the naked eye. Colonies of cells that have been transformed by a successfully recombined plasmid will thus appear white whereas those that have been transformed by non-recombined plasmid will appear blue.

Plants

A number of mechanisms are available to transfer DNA into plant cells:

- *Agrobacterium* mediated transformation is the easiest and most simple plant transformation. Plant tissue (often leaves) are cut into small pieces, e.g. 10x10mm, and soaked for 10 minutes in a fluid containing suspended *Agrobacterium*. Some cells along the cut will be transformed by the bacterium, that inserts its DNA into the cell. Placed on selectable rooting and shooting media, the plants will regrow. Some plants species can be transformed just by dipping the flowers into suspension of *Agrobacterium* and then planting the seeds in a selective medium. Unfortunately, many plants are not transformable by this method.
- Particle bombardment: Particles of gold or tungsten are coated with DNA and then shot into young plant cells or plant embryos.

Some genetic material will stay in the cells and transform them. This method also allows transformation of plant plastids. The transformation efficiency is lower than in agribacterial mediated transformation, but most plants can be transformed with this method.

- Electroporation: make transient holes in cell membranes using electric shock; this allows DNA to enter as described above for Bacteria.
- Viral transformation (transduction): Package the desired genetic material into a suitable plant virus and allow this modified virus to infect the plant. If the genetic material is DNA, it can recombine with the chromosomes to produce transformant cells. However genomes of most plant viruses consist of single stranded RNA which replicates in the cytoplasm of infected cell. For such genomes this method is a form of transfection and not a real transformation, since the inserted genes never reach the nucleus of the cell and do not integrate into the host genome. The progeny of the infected plants is virus free and also free of the inserted gene.

Animals

Introduction of DNA into animal cells is usually called transfection, and is discussed in the corresponding article.

Selection

Not all the organism's cells will be transformed with the new genetic material; in most cases a selectable marker is used to differentiate transformed from untransformed cells. If a cell has been successfully transformed with the DNA it will also contain the marker gene. By growing the cells in the presence of an antibiotic or chemical that selects or marks the cells expressing that gene it is possible to separate the transgenic events from the non-transgenic. Another method of screening involves using a DNA probe that will only stick to the inserted gene. A number of strategies have been developed that can remove the selectable marker from the mature transgenic plant.

Regeneration

As often only a single cell is transformed with genetic material the organism must be regrown from that single cell. As bacteria consist of a single cell and reproduce clonally regeneration is not necessary. In plants this is accomplished through the use of tissue culture. Each plant species has different requirements for successful regeneration through tissue culture. If successful an adult plant is produced that contains the transgene in every cell. In animals it is necessary to ensure that the inserted DNA is present in the embryonic stem cells. When the offspring is produced they can be screened for the presence of the gene. All offspring from the first generation will be heterozygous for the inserted gene and must be mated together to produce a homozygous animal.

Confirmation

Further tests using PCR, Southern Blots and Bioassays are needed to confirm that the gene is expressed and functions correctly. The organism's offspring are also tested to ensure that the trait can be inherited and that it follows a Mendelian inheritance pattern.

Applications

Genetic engineering has applications in medicine, research, industry and agriculture and can be used on a wide range of plants, animals and micro organism.

Medicine

In medicine genetic engineering has been used to mass produce insulin, human growth hormones, follistim (for treating infertility), human albumin, monoclonal antibodies, antihemophilic factors, vaccines and many other drugs. Vaccination generally involves injecting weak live, killed or inactivated forms of viruses or their toxins into the person being immunized. Genetically engineered viruses are being developed that can still confer immunity, but lack the infectious sequences. Mouse hybridomas, cells fused together to create monoclonal antibodies, have been humanised through genetic engineering to create human monoclonal antibodies.

Genetic engineering is used to create animal models of human diseases. Genetically modified mice are the most common genetically engineered animal model. They have been used to study and model cancer (the oncomouse), obesity, heart disease, diabetes, arthritis, substance abuse, anxiety, aging and Parkinson disease. Potential cures can be tested against these mouse models. Also genetically modified pigs have been bred with the aim of increasing the success of pig to human organ transplantation.

Gene therapy is the genetic engineering of humans by replacing defective human genes with functional copies. This can occur in somatic tissue or germline tissue. If the gene is inserted into the germline tissue it can be passed down to that person's descendants. Gene therapy has been used to treat patients suffering from immune deficiencies (notably Severe combined immunodeficiency) and trials have been carried out on other genetic disorders. The success of gene therapy so far has been limited and a patient (Jesse Gelsinger) has died during a clinical trial testing a new treatment. There are also ethical concerns should the technology be used not just for treatment, but for enhancement, modification or alteration of a human beings' appearance, adaptability, intelligence, character or Behaviour. The distinction between cure and enhancement can also be difficult to establish. Transhumanists consider the enhancement of humans desirable.

Research

Genetic engineering is an important tool for natural scientists. Genes and other genetic information from a wide range of organisms are transformed into bacteria for storage and modification, creating genetically modified bacteria in the process. Bacteria are cheap, easy to grow, clonal, multiply quickly, relatively easy to transform and can be stored at -80°C almost indefinitely. Once a gene is isolated it can be stored inside the bacteria providing an unlimited supply for research.

Organisms are genetically engineered to discover the functions of certain genes. This could be the effect on the phenotype of the organism, where the gene is expressed or what other genes it interacts with. These experiments generally involve loss of function, gain of function, tracking and expression.

- Loss of function experiments, such as in a gene knockout experiment, in which an organism is engineered to lack the activity of one or more genes. A knockout experiment involves the creation and manipulation of a DNA construct *in vitro*, which, in a simple knockout, consists of a copy of the desired gene, which has been altered such that it is non-functional. Embryonic stem cells incorporate the altered gene, which replaces the already present functional copy. These stem cells are injected into blastocysts, which are implanted into surrogate mothers. This allows the experimenter to analyse the defects caused by this mutation and thereby determine the role of particular genes. It is used especially frequently in developmental biology. Another method, useful in organisms such as Drosophila (fruit fly), is to induce mutations in a large population and then screen the progeny for the desired mutation. A similar process can be used in both plants and prokaryotes.

- Gain of function experiments, the logical counterpart of knockouts. These are sometimes performed in conjunction with knockout experiments to more finely establish the function of the desired gene. The process is much the same as that in knockout engineering, except that the construct is designed to increase the function of the gene, usually by providing extra copies of the gene or inducing synthesis of the protein more frequently.
- Tracking experiments, which seek to gain information about the localization and interaction of the desired protein. One way to do this is to replace the wild-type gene with a 'fusion' gene, which is a juxtaposition of the wild-type gene with a reporting element such as green fluorescent protein (GFP) that will allow easy visualization of the products of the genetic modification. While this is a useful technique, the manipulation can destroy the function of the gene, creating secondary effects and possibly calling into question the results of the experiment. More sophisticated techniques are now in development that can track protein products without mitigating their function, such as the addition of small sequences that will serve as binding motifs to monoclonal antibodies.
- Expression studies aim to discover where and when specific proteins are produced. In these experiments, the DNA sequence before the DNA that codes for a protein, known as a gene's promoter, is reintroduced into an organism with the protein coding region replaced by a reporter gene such as GFP or an enzyme that catalyses the production of a dye. Thus the time and place where a particular protein is produced can be observed. Expression studies can be taken a step further by altering the promoter to find which pieces are crucial for the proper expression of the gene and are actually bound by transcription factor proteins; this process is known as promoter bashing.

Industrial

By engineering genes into bacterial plasmids it is possible to create a biological factory that can produce proteins and enzymes. Some genes do not work well in bacteria, so yeast, a eukaryote, can also be used.

Bacteria and yeast factories have been used to produce medicines such as insulin, human growth hormone, and vaccines, supplements such as tryptophan, aid in the production of food (chymosin in cheese making) and fuels. Other applications involving genetically engineered bacteria being investigated involve making the bacteria perform tasks outside their natural cycle, such as cleaning up oil spills, carbon and other toxic waste.

Agriculture

One of the best-known and controversial applications of genetic engineering is the creation of genetically modified food. There are three generations of genetically modified crops. First generation crops have been commercialized and most provide protection from insects and/or resistance to herbicides. There are also fungal and virus resistant crops developed or in development. They have been developed to make the insect and weed management of crops easier and can indirectly increase crop yield.

The second generation of genetically modified crops being developed aim to directly improve yield by improving salt, cold or drought tolerance and to increase the nutritional value of the crops. The third generation consists of pharmaceutical crops, crops that contain edible vaccines and other drugs. Some agriculturally important animals have been genetically modified with growth hormones to increase their size while others have been engineered to express drugs and other proteins in their milk.

The genetic engineering of agricultural crops can increase the growth rates and resistance to different diseases caused by pathogens and parasites. This is beneficial as it can greatly increase the production of food sources with the usage of fewer resources that would be required to host the world's growing populations. These modified crops would also reduce the usage of chemicals, such as fertilizers and pesticides, and therefore decrease the severity and frequency of the damages produced by these chemical pollution.

Ethical and safety concerns have been raised around the use of genetically modified food. A major safety concern relates to the human health implications of eating genetically modified food, in particular whether toxic or allergic reactions could occur. Gene flow into related non-transgenic crops, off target effects on beneficial organisms and the impact on biodiversity are important environmental issues. Ethical concerns involve religious issues, corporate control of the food supply, intellectual property rights and the level of labeling needed on genetically modified products.

Other uses

In materials science, a genetically modified virus has been used to construct a more environmentally friendly lithium-ion battery. Some bacteria have been genetically engineered to create black and white photographs while others have potential to be used as sensors by expressing a fluorescent protein under certain environmental conditions. Genetic engineering is also being used to create BioArt and novelty items such as blue roses, and glowing fish.

Opposition and Criticism

A 2010 study of Canola found transgenes in 80% of wild (uncultivated or "feral") varieties in North Dakota, meaning 80% of the plants which had established themselves in the area were genetically engineered varieties. The researchers stated that "we found the highest densities of [such transgene-containing] plants near agricultural fields and along major freeways, but we were also finding plants in the middle of nowhere" adding that "over time,..the build-up of different types of herbicide resistance in feral [natural] canola and closely related weeds, like field mustard, could make it more difficult to manage these plants using herbicides."

Selection

Not all the organism's cells will be transformed with the new genetic material; in most cases a selectable marker is used to differentiate transformed from untransformed cells. If a cell has been successfully transformed with the DNA it will also contain the marker gene. By growing the cells in the presence of an antibiotic or chemical that selects or marks the cells expressing that gene it is possible to separate the transgenic events from the non-transgenic. Another method of screening involves using a DNA probe that will only stick to the inserted gene. A number of strategies have been developed that can remove the selectable marker from the mature transgenic plant.

Regeneration

As often only a single cell is transformed with genetic material the organism must be regrown from that single cell. As bacteria consist of a single cell and reproduce clonally regeneration is not necessary. In plants this is accomplished through the use of tissue culture. Each plant species has different requirements for successful regeneration through tissue culture. If successful an adult plant is produced that contains the transgene in every cell. In animals it is necessary to ensure that the inserted DNA is present in the embryonic stem cells. When the offspring is produced they can be screened for the presence of the gene. All offspring from the first generation will be heterozygous for the inserted gene and must be mated together to produce a homozygous animal.

Confirmation

Further tests using PCR, Southern Blots and Bioassays are needed to confirm that the gene is expressed and functions correctly. The organism's offspring are also tested to ensure that the trait can be inherited and that it follows a Mendelian inheritance pattern.

Applications

Genetic engineering has applications in medicine, research, industry and agriculture and can be used on a wide range of plants, animals and micro organism.

Medicine

In medicine genetic engineering has been used to mass produce insulin, human growth hormones, follistim (for treating infertility), human albumin, monoclonal antibodies, antihemophilic factors, vaccines and many other drugs. Vaccination generally involves injecting weak live, killed or inactivated forms of viruses or their toxins into the person being immunized. Genetically engineered viruses are being developed that can still confer immunity, but lack the infectious sequences. Mouse hybridomas, cells fused together to create monoclonal antibodies, have been humanised through genetic engineering to create human monoclonal antibodies.

Genetic engineering is used to create animal models of human diseases. Genetically modified mice are the most common genetically engineered animal model. They have been used to study and model cancer (the oncomouse), obesity, heart disease, diabetes, arthritis, substance abuse, anxiety, aging and Parkinson disease. Potential cures can be tested against these mouse models. Also genetically modified pigs have been bred with the aim of increasing the success of pig to human organ transplantation.

Gene therapy is the genetic engineering of humans by replacing defective human genes with functional copies. This can occur in somatic tissue or germline tissue. If the gene is inserted into the germline tissue it can be passed down to that person's descendants. Gene therapy has been used to treat patients suffering from immune deficiencies (notably Severe combined immunodeficiency) and trials have been carried out on other genetic disorders. The success of gene therapy so far has been limited and a patient (Jesse Gelsinger) has died during a clinical trial testing a new treatment. There are also ethical concerns should the technology be used not just for treatment, but for enhancement, modification or alteration of a human beings' appearance, adaptability, intelligence, character or Behaviour. The distinction between cure and enhancement can also be difficult to establish. Transhumanists consider the enhancement of humans desirable.

Research

Genetic engineering is an important tool for natural scientists. Genes and other genetic information from a wide range of organisms are transformed into bacteria for storage and modification, creating genetically modified bacteria in the process. Bacteria are cheap, easy to grow, clonal, multiply quickly, relatively easy to transform and can be stored at -80°C almost indefinitely. Once a gene is isolated it can be stored inside the bacteria providing an unlimited supply for research.

Organisms are genetically engineered to discover the functions of certain genes. This could be the effect on the phenotype of the organism, where the gene is expressed or what other genes it interacts with. These experiments generally involve loss of function, gain of function, tracking and expression.

- Loss of function experiments, such as in a gene knockout experiment, in which an organism is engineered to lack the activity of one or more genes. A knockout experiment involves the creation and manipulation of a DNA construct *in vitro*, which, in a simple knockout, consists of a copy of the desired gene, which has been altered such that it is non-functional. Embryonic stem cells incorporate the altered gene, which replaces the already present functional copy. These stem cells are injected into blastocysts, which are implanted into surrogate mothers. This allows the experimenter to analyse the defects caused by this mutation and thereby determine the role of particular genes. It is used especially frequently in developmental biology. Another method, useful in organisms such as Drosophila (fruit fly), is to induce mutations in a large population and then screen the progeny for the desired mutation. A similar process can be used in both plants and prokaryotes.
- Gain of function experiments, the logical counterpart of knockouts. These are sometimes performed in conjunction with

knockout experiments to more finely establish the function of the desired gene. The process is much the same as that in knockout engineering, except that the construct is designed to increase the function of the gene, usually by providing extra copies of the gene or inducing synthesis of the protein more frequently.

- Tracking experiments, which seek to gain information about the localization and interaction of the desired protein. One way to do this is to replace the wild-type gene with a 'fusion' gene, which is a juxtaposition of the wild-type gene with a reporting element such as green fluorescent protein (GFP) that will allow easy visualization of the products of the genetic modification. While this is a useful technique, the manipulation can destroy the function of the gene, creating secondary effects and possibly calling into question the results of the experiment. More sophisticated techniques are now in development that can track protein products without mitigating their function, such as the addition of small sequences that will serve as binding motifs to monoclonal antibodies.
- Expression studies aim to discover where and when specific proteins are produced. In these experiments, the DNA sequence before the DNA that codes for a protein, known as a gene's promoter, is reintroduced into an organism with the protein coding region replaced by a reporter gene such as GFP or an enzyme that catalyses the production of a dye. Thus the time and place where a particular protein is produced can be observed. Expression studies can be taken a step further by altering the promoter to find which pieces are crucial for the proper expression of the gene and are actually bound by transcription factor proteins; this process is known as promoter bashing.

Industrial

By engineering genes into bacterial plasmids it is possible to create a biological factory that can produce proteins and enzymes. Some genes do not work well in bacteria, so yeast, a eukaryote, can also be used. Bacteria and yeast factories have been used to produce medicines such as insulin, human growth hormone, and vaccines, supplements such as tryptophan, aid in the production of food (chymosin in cheese making) and fuels. Other applications involving genetically engineered bacteria being investigated involve making the bacteria perform tasks outside their natural cycle, such as cleaning up oil spills, carbon and other toxic waste.

Agriculture

One of the best-known and controversial applications of genetic engineering is the creation of genetically modified food. There are three generations of genetically modified crops. First generation crops have been commercialized and most provide protection from insects and/or resistance to herbicides. There are also fungal and virus resistant crops developed or in development. They have been developed to make the insect and weed management of crops easier and can indirectly increase crop yield.

The second generation of genetically modified crops being developed aim to directly improve yield by improving salt, cold or drought tolerance and to increase the nutritional value of the crops. The third generation consists of pharmaceutical crops, crops that contain edible vaccines and other drugs. Some agriculturally important animals have been genetically modified with growth hormones to increase their size while others have been engineered to express drugs and other proteins in their milk.

The genetic engineering of agricultural crops can increase the growth rates and resistance to different diseases caused by pathogens and parasites. This is beneficial as it can greatly increase the production of food sources with the usage of fewer resources that would be required to host the world's growing populations. These modified crops would also reduce the usage of chemicals, such as fertilizers and pesticides, and therefore decrease the severity and frequency of the damages produced by these chemical pollution.

Ethical and safety concerns have been raised around the use of genetically modified food. A major safety concern relates to the human health implications of eating genetically modified food, in particular whether toxic or allergic reactions could occur. Gene flow into related non-transgenic crops, off target effects on beneficial organisms and the impact on biodiversity are important environmental issues. Ethical concerns involve religious issues, corporate control of the food supply, intellectual property rights and the level of labeling needed on genetically modified products.

Other Uses

In materials science, a genetically modified virus has been used to construct a more environmentally friendly lithium-ion battery.

Some bacteria have been genetically engineered to create black and white photographs while others have potential to be used as sensors by expressing a fluorescent protein under certain environmental conditions. Genetic engineering is also being used to create BioArt and novelty items such as blue roses, and glowing fish.

Opposition and Criticism

A 2010 study of Canola found transgenes in 80% of wild (uncultivated or "feral") varieties in North Dakota, meaning 80% of the plants which had established themselves in the area were genetically engineered varieties. The researchers stated that "we found the highest densities of [such transgene-containing] plants near agricultural fields and along major freeways, but we were also finding plants in the middle of nowhere" adding that "over time,..the build-up of different types of herbicide resistance in feral [natural] canola and closely related weeds, like field mustard, could make it more difficult to manage these plants using herbicides."

DNA Profiling

DNA profiling (also called DNA testing, DNA typing, or genetic fingerprinting) is a technique employed by forensic scientists to assist in the identification of individuals by their respective DNA profiles. DNA profiles are encrypted sets of numbers that reflect a person's DNA makeup, which can also be used as the person's identifier. DNA profiling should not be confused with full genome sequencing. It is used in, for example, parental testing and rape investigation.

Although 99.9% of human DNA sequences are the same in every person, enough of the DNA is different to distinguish one individual from another. DNA profiling uses repetitive ("repeat") sequences that are highly variable, called variable number tandem repeats (VNTR). VNTRs loci are very similar between closely related humans, but so variable that unrelated individuals are extremely unlikely to have the same VNTRs.

The DNA profiling technique was first reported in 1984 by Sir Alec Jeffreys at the University of Leicester in England, and is now the basis of several national DNA databases. Dr. Jeffreys's genetic fingerprinting was made commercially available in 1987, when a chemical company, ICI, started a blood-testing centre in England.

DNA Profiling Process

The process begins with a sample of an individual's DNA (typically called a "reference sample"). The most desirable method of collecting a reference sample is the use of a buccal swab, as this reduces the possibility of contamination. When this is not available (e.g. because a court order may be needed and not obtainable) other methods may need to be used to collect a sample of blood, saliva, semen, or other appropriate fluid or tissue from personal items (e.g. toothbrush, razor, etc.) or from stored samples (e.g. banked sperm or biopsy tissue). Samples obtained from blood relatives (biological relative) can provide an indication of an individual's profile, as could human remains which had been previously profiled.

A reference sample is then analysed to create the individual's DNA profile using one of a number of techniques, discussed below. The DNA profile is then compared against another sample to determine whether there is a genetic match.

Restriction Fragment Length Polymorphism

In molecular biology, the term restriction fragment length polymorphism, or RFLP, (commonly pronounced "rif-lip") is a technique that exploits variations in homologous DNA sequences. It refers to a difference between samples of homologous DNA molecules that come from differing locations of restriction enzyme sites, and to a related laboratory technique by which these segments can be illustrated.

In RFLP analysis the DNA sample is broken into pieces (digested) by restriction enzymes and the resulting *restriction fragments* are separated according to their lengths by gel electrophoresis. Although now largely obsolete, RFLP analysis was the first DNA profiling technique inexpensive enough to see widespread application. In addition to genetic fingerprinting, RFLP was an important tool in genome mapping, localization of genes for genetic disorders, determination of risk for disease, and paternity testing.

Analysis Technique

The basic technique for detecting RFLPs involves fragmenting a sample of DNA by a restriction enzyme, which can recognize and cut DNA wherever a specific short sequence occurs, in a process known as a restriction digest.

The resulting DNA fragments are then separated by length through a process known as agarose gel electrophoresis, and transferred to a membrane via the Southern blot procedure. Hybridization of the membrane to a labelled DNA probe then determines the length of the fragments which are complementary to the probe. An RFLP occurs when the length of a detected fragment varies between individuals. Each fragment length is considered an allele, and can be used in genetic analysis.

RFLP analysis may be subdivided into single- (SLP) and multi-locus probe (MLP) paradigms. Usually, the SLP method is preferred over MLP because it is more sensitive, easier to interpret and capable of analyzing mixed-DNA samples. Moreover data can be generated even when the DNA is degraded (e.g. when it is found in bone remains.)

Examples

There are two common mechanisms by which the size of a particular restriction fragment can vary. In the first schematic, a small segment of the genome is being detected by a DNA probe (thicker line). In allele "A", the genome is cleaved by a restriction enzyme at three nearby sites (triangles), but only the rightmost fragment will be detected by the probe. In allele "a", restriction site 2 has been lost by a mutation, so the probe now detects the larger fused fragment running from sites 1 to 3. The second diagram shows how this fragment size variation would look on a Southern blot, and how each allele (two per individual) might be inherited in members of a family.

In the third schematic, the probe and restriction enzyme are chosen to detect a region of the genome that includes a variable VNTR segment (boxes). In allele "c" there are five repeats in the VNTR, and the probe detects a longer fragment between the two restriction sites. In allele "d" there are only two repeats in the VNTR, so the probe detects a shorter fragment between the same two restriction sites. Other genetic processes, such as insertions, deletions, translocations, and inversions, can also lead to RFLPs.

Applications

Analysis of RFLP variation in genomes was a vital tool in genome mapping and genetic disease analysis. If researchers were trying to initially determine the chromosomal location of a particular disease gene, they would analyse the DNA of members of a family afflicted by the disease, and look for RFLP alleles that show a similar pattern of inheritance as that of the disease. Once a disease gene was localized, RFLP analysis of other families could reveal who was at risk for the disease, or who was likely to be carriers of the mutant genes.

RFLP analysis was also the basis for early methods of Genetic fingerprinting, useful in the identification of samples retrieved from crime scenes, in the determination of paternity, and in the characterization of genetic diversity or breeding patterns in animal populations.

Alternatives

The technique for RFLP analysis is, however, slow and cumbersome. It requires a large amount of sample DNA, and the combined process of probe labeling, DNA fragmentation, electrophoresis, blotting, hybridization, washing, and autoradiography could take up to a month to complete. A limited version of the RFLP method that used oligonucleotide probes was reported in 1985. Fortunately, the results of the Human Genome Project have largely replaced the need for RFLP mapping, and the identification of many single-nucleotide polymorphisms (SNPs) in that project (as well as the direct identification of many disease genes and mutations) has replaced the need for RFLP disease linkage analysis. The analysis of VNTR alleles continues, but is now usually performed by polymerase chain reaction (PCR) methods. For example, the standard protocols for DNA fingerprinting involve PCR analysis of panels of more than a dozen VNTRs.

RFLP is still a technique used in marker assisted selection. Terminal restriction fragment length polymorphism (TRFLP or sometimes T-RFLP) is a molecular biology technique initially developed for characterizing bacterial communities in mixed-species samples. The technique has also been applied to other groups including soil fungi.

TRFLP works by PCR amplification of DNA using primer pairs that have been labelled with fluorescent tags. The PCR products are then digested using RFLP enzymes and the resulting patterns visualized using a DNA sequencer. The results are analysed either by simply counting and comparing bands or peaks in the TRFLP profile, or by matching bands from one or more TRFLP runs to a database of known species. The technique is similar in some aspects to DGGE or TGGE.

The sequence changes directly involved with an RFLP can also be analysed more quickly by PCR. Amplification can be directed across the altered restriction site, and the products digested with the restriction enzyme. This method has been called Cleaved Amplified Polymorphic Sequence (CAPS). Alternatively, the amplified segment can by analysed by Allele specific oligonucleotide (ASO) probes, a process that can often be done by a simple Dot blot.

Short Tandem Repeat

A short tandem repeat (STR) in DNA occurs when a pattern of two or more nucleotides are repeated and the repeated sequences are directly adjacent to each other. The pattern can range in length from 2 to 50 base pairs (bp) (for example $(CATG)_n$ in a genomic region) and is typically in the non-coding intron region. A short tandem repeat polymorphism (STRP) occurs when homologous STR loci differ in the number of repeats between individuals.

By identifying repeats of a specific sequence at specific locations in the genome, it is possible to create a genetic profile of an individual. There are currently over 10,000 published STR sequences in the human genome. STR analysis has become the prevalent analysis method for determining genetic profiles in forensic cases.

Forensic STR Analysis

STR analysis is a relatively new technology in the field of forensics, having come into popularity in the mid-to-late 1990s. It is used for the genetic fingerprinting of individuals. The STRs in use today for forensic analysis are all tetra- or penta-nucleotide repeats (4 or 5 repeated nucleotides), as these give a high degree of error-free data while being robust enough to survive degradation in non-ideal conditions. Shorter repeat sequences tend to suffer from artifacts such as PCR stutter and preferential amplification, as well as the fact that several genetic diseases are associated with tri-nucleotide repeats such as Huntington's disease. Longer repeat sequences will suffer more highly from environmental degradation and do not amplify by PCR as well as shorter sequences.

The analysis is performed by extracting nuclear DNA from the cells of a forensic sample of interest, then amplifying specific polymorphic regions of the extracted DNA by means of the polymerase chain reaction. Once these sequences have been amplified, they are resolved either through gel electrophoresis or capillary electrophoresis, which will allow the analyst to determine how many repeats of the STR sequence in question there are. If the DNA was resolved by gel electrophoresis, the DNA can be visualized either by silver staining (not very high resolution, safe, inexpensive), or an intercalating dye such as ethidium bromide (fairly sensitive, moderate health risks, inexpensive), or as most modern forensics labs use, fluorescent dyes (highly sensitive, safe, expensive).

Instruments built to resolve STR fragments by capillary electrophoresis also use fluorescent dyes to great effect. It is also used to follow up bone marrow transplant patients. In the United States, 13 core STR loci have been decided upon to be the basis by which an individual genetic profile can be generated.

These profiles are stored on a local, state and national level in DNA databanks such as CODIS. The British data base for STR loci identification is the UK National DNA Database (NDNAD). The British system uses 10 loci, rather than the American 13 loci.

Y-STRs (STRs on the Y chromosome) are often used in genealogical DNA testing.

Amplified Fragment Length Polymorphism

Amplified Fragment Length Polymorphism PCR (or AFLP-PCR or just AFLP) is a PCR-based tool used in genetics research, DNA fingerprinting, and in the practice of genetic engineering. Developed in the early 1990s by Keygene, AFLP uses restriction enzymes to digest genomic DNA, followed by ligation of adaptors to the sticky ends of the restriction fragments. A subset of the restriction fragments is then selected to be amplified.

This selection is achieved by using primers complementary to the adaptor sequence, the restriction site sequence and a few nucleotides inside the restriction site fragments (as described in detail below). The amplified fragments are visualized on denaturing polyacrylamide gels either through autoradiography or fluorescence methodologies.

AFLP-PCR is a highly sensitive method for detecting polymorphisms in DNA. The technique was originally described by Vos and Zabeau in 1993. In detail, the procedure of this technique is divided into three steps:

1. Digestion of total cellular DNA with one or more restriction enzymes and ligation of restriction half-site specific adaptors to all restriction fragments.
2. Selective amplification of some of these fragments with two PCR primers that have corresponding adaptor and restriction site specific sequences.
3. Electrophoretic separation of amplicons on a gel matrix, followed by visualisation of the band pattern.

A variation on AFLP is cDNA-AFLP, which is used to quantify differences in gene expression levels.

Another variation on AFLP is TE Display, used to detect transposable element mobility.

Applications

The AFLP technology has the capability to detect various polymorphisms in different genomic regions simultaneously. It is also highly sensitive and reproducible. As a result, AFLP has become widely used for the identification of genetic variation in strains or closely related species of plants, fungi, animals, and bacteria. The AFLP technology has been used in criminal and paternity tests, also to determine slight differences within populations, and in linkage studies to generate maps for quantitative trait locus (QTL) analysis.

There are many advantages to AFLP when compared to other marker technologies including randomly amplified polymorphic DNA (RAPD), restriction fragment length polymorphism (RFLP), and microsatellites. AFLP not only has higher reproducibility, resolution, and sensitivity at the whole genome level compared to other techniques, but it also has the capability to amplify between 50 and 100 fragments at one time. In addition, no prior sequence information is needed for amplification (Meudt & Clarke 2007). As a result, AFLP has become extremely beneficial in the study of taxa including bacteria, fungi, and plants, where much is still unknown about the genomic makeup of various organisms.

The AFLP technology is covered by patents and patent applications of Keygene N.V. AFLP is a registered trademark of Keygene N.V.

DNA Family Relationship Analysis

Using PCR technology, DNA analysis is widely applied to determine genetic family relationships such as paternity, maternity, siblingship and other kinships.

During conception, the father's sperm cell and the mother's egg cell, each containing half the amount of DNA found in other body cells, meet and fuse to form a fertilized egg, called a zygote. The zygote contains a complete set of DNA molecules, a unique combination of DNA from both parents. This zygote divides and multiplies into an embryo and later, a full human being.

At each stage of development, all the cells forming the body contain the same DNA—half from the father and half from the mother. This fact allows the relationship testing to use all types of all samples including loose cells from the cheeks collected using buccal swabs, blood or other types of samples.

While a lot of DNA contains information for a certain function, there is some called junk DNA, which is currently used for human identification. At some special locations (called loci) in the junk DNA, predictable inheritance patterns were found to be useful in determining biological relationships.

These locations contain specific DNA markers that DNA scientists use to identify individuals. In a routine DNA paternity test, the markers used are Short Tandem Repeats (STRs), short pieces of DNA that occur in highly differential repeat patterns among individuals.

Each person's DNA contains two copies of these markers—one copy inherited from the father and one from the mother. Within a population, the markers at each person's DNA location could differ in length and sometimes sequence, depending on the markers inherited from the parents.

The combination of marker sizes found in each person makes up his/her unique genetic profile. When determining the relationship between two individuals, their genetic profiles are compared to see if they share the same inheritance patterns at a statistically conclusive rate.

For example, the following sample report from this commercial DNA paternity testing laboratory Universal Genetics signifies how relatedness between parents and child is identified on those special markers:

DNA Marker	*Mother*	*Child*	*Alleged father*
D21S11	28, 30	28, 31	29, 31
D7S820	9, 10	10, 11	11, 12
TH01	14, 15	14, 16	15, 16
D13S317	7, 8	7, 9	8, 9
D19S433	14, 16.2	14, 15	15, 17

The partial results indicate that the child and the alleged father's DNA match among these five markers. The complete test results show this correlation on 16 markers between the child and the tested man to draw a conclusion of whether or not the man is the biological father.

Scientifically, each marker is assigned with a Paternity Index (PI), which is a statistical measure of how powerfully a match at a particular marker indicates paternity.

The PI of each marker is multiplied with each other to generate the Combined Paternity Index (CPI), which indicates the overall probability of an individual being the biological father of the tested child relative to any random man from the entire population of the same race.

The CPI is then converted into a Probability of Paternity showing the degree of relatedness between the alleged father and child.

The DNA test report in other family relationship tests, such as grandparentage and siblingship tests, is similar to a paternity test report. Instead of the Combined Paternity Index, a different value, such as a Siblingship Index, is reported.

The report shows the genetic profiles of each tested person. If there are markers shared among the tested individuals, the probability of biological relationship is calculated to determine how likely the tested individuals share the same markers due to a blood relationship.

Y-chromosome Analysis

Recent innovations have included the creation of primers targeting polymorphic regions on the Y-chromosome (Y-STR), which allows resolution of a mixed DNA sample from a male and female and/or cases in which a differential extraction is not possible. Y-chromosomes are paternally inherited, so Y-STR analysis can help in the identification of paternally related males. Y-STR analysis was performed in the Sally Hemings controversy to determine if Thomas Jefferson had sired a son with one of his slaves.

Mitochondrial DNA

Replication

mtDNA is replicated by the DNA polymerase gamma complex which is composed of a 140 kDa catalytic DNA polymerase encoded by the *POLG* gene and a 55 kDa accessory subunit encoded by the *POLG2* gene. During embryogenesis, replication of mtDNA is strictly down-regulated from the fertilized oocyte through the preimplantation embryo. At the blastocyst stage, the onset of mtDNA replication is specific to the cells of the trophectoderm. In contrast, the cells of the inner cell mass restrict mtDNA replication until they receive the signals to differentiate to specific cell types.

Origin

Nuclear and mitochondrial DNA are thought to be of separate evolutionary origin, with the mtDNA being derived from the circular genomes of the bacteria that were engulfed by the early ancestors of today's eukaryotic cells. This theory is called the endosymbiotic theory.

Each mitochondrion is estimated to contain 2-10 mtDNA copies. In the cells of extant organisms, the vast majority of the proteins present in the mitochondria (numbering approximately 1500 different types in mammals) are coded for by nuclear DNA, but the genes for some of them, if not most, are thought to have originally been of bacterial origin, having since been transferred to the eukaryotic nucleus during evolution.

Mitochondrial Inheritance

In most multicellular organisms, mtDNA is inherited from the mother (maternally inherited). Mechanisms for this include simple dilution (an egg contains 100,000 to 1,000,000 mtDNA molecules, whereas a sperm contains only 100 to 1000), degradation of sperm mtDNA in the fertilized egg, and, at least in a few organisms, failure of sperm mtDNA to enter the egg. Whatever the mechanism, this single parent (uniparental) pattern of mtDNA inheritance is found in most animals, most plants and in fungi as well.

Female Inheritance

In sexual reproduction, mitochondria are normally inherited exclusively from the mother. The mitochondria in mammalian sperm are usually destroyed by the egg cell after fertilization. Also, most mitochondria are present at the base of the sperm's tail, which is used for propelling the sperm cells. Sometimes the tail is lost during fertilization. In 1999 it was reported that paternal sperm mitochondria (containing mtDNA) are marked with ubiquitin to select them for later destruction inside the embryo. Some *in vitro* fertilization techniques, particularly injecting a sperm into an oocyte, may interfere with this.

The fact that mitochondrial DNA is maternally inherited enables researchers to trace maternal lineage far back in time. (Y chromosomal DNA, paternally inherited, is used in an analogous way to trace the agnate lineage.) This is accomplished in humans by sequencing one or more of the hypervariable control regions (HVR1 or HVR2) of the mitochondrial DNA, as with a genealogical DNA test. HVR1 consists of about 440 base pairs. These 440 base pairs are then compared to the control regions of other individuals (either specific people or subjects in a database) to determine maternal lineage. Most often, the comparison is made to the revised Cambridge Reference Sequence. Vilà *et al.* have published studies tracing the matrilineal descent of domestic dogs to wolves. The concept of the Mitochondrial Eve is based on the same type of analysis, attempting to discover the origin of humanity by tracking the lineage back in time.

Because mtDNA is not highly conserved and has a rapid mutation rate, it is useful for studying the evolutionary relationships - phylogeny

- of organisms. Biologists can determine and then compare mtDNA sequences among different species and use the comparisons to build an evolutionary tree for the species examined.

Because mtDNA is transmitted from mother to child (both male and female), it can be a useful tool in genealogical research into a person's maternal line.

Paternal mtDNA Transmission

In genetics, paternal mtDNA transmission and paternal mtDNA inheritance refer to the incidence of mitochondrial DNA (mtDNA) being passed from a father to his offspring. Paternal mtDNA inheritance is observed in a small proportion of species; in general, mtDNA is passed unchanged from a mother to her offspring, making it an example of non-Mendelian inheritance. In contrast, mtDNA transmission from both parents occurs regularly in certain bivalves.

In Animals

Paternal mtDNA inheritance in animals varies. For example, in Mytilidae mussels, paternal mtDNA "is transmitted through the sperm and establishes itself only in the male gonad." In testing 172 sheep, "The Mitochondrial DNA from three lambs in two half-sib families were found to show paternal inheritance."

In Humans

In human mitochondrial genetics, there is debate over whether or not paternal mtDNA transmission is possible. Many studies hold that paternal mtDNA is never transmitted to offspring. This belief is central to mtDNA genealogical DNA testing and to the theory of mitochondrial Eve. The fact that mitochondrial DNA is maternally inherited enables researchers to trace maternal lineage far back in time. (Y chromosomal DNA, paternally inherited, is used in an analogous way to trace the agnate lineage.)

In sexual reproduction, paternal mitochondria found in the sperm are actively decomposed, thus preventing "paternal leakage". Mitochondria in mammalian sperm are usually destroyed by the egg cell after fertilization. In 1999 it was reported that paternal sperm mitochondria (containing mtDNA) are marked with ubiquitin to select them for later destruction inside the embryo. Some in vitro fertilization (IVF) techniques, particularly intracytoplasmic sperm injection (ICSI) of a sperm into an oocyte, may interfere with this.

It is now understood that the tail of the sperm, which contains additional mtDNA, may also enter the egg. This had led to increased controversy about the fate of paternal mtDNA.

Some sources state that so little paternal mtDNA is transmitted as to be negligible ("At most, one presumes it must be less than 1 in 1000, since there are 100 000 mitochondria in the human egg and only 100 in the sperm (Satoh and Kuroiwa, 1991).") or that paternal mtDNA is so rarely transmitted as to be negligible ("Nevertheless, studies have established that paternal mtDNA is so rarely transmitted to offspring that mtDNA analyses remain valid..."). One study stated that about 1–2% of a person's mitochondria can be inherited from the father.

The controversy about human paternal leakage was summed up in the 1996 study *Misconceptions about mitochondria and mammalian fertilization: Implications for theories on human evolution.* The following quotation comes from the abstract to that peer-reviewed study printed in the *Proceedings of the National Academy of Sciences*: The mixing of maternal and paternal mtDNA was thought to have been found in humans and chimpanzees in 1999. However, there has been only a single documented case of human paternal mitochondrial DNA transmission, and it was linked to infertility.

According to the 2005 study *More evidence for non-maternal inheritance of mitochondrial DNA?*, heteroplasmy is a "newly discovered form of inheritance for mtDNA. Heteroplasmy introduces slight statistical uncertainty in normal inheritance patterns." Heteroplasmy may result from a mutation during development which is propagated to only a subset of the adult cells, or may occur when two slightly different mitochondrial sequences are inherited from the mother as a result of several hundred mitochondria being present in the ovum.

In Protozoa

Some organisms, such as *Cryptosporidium*, have mitochondria with no DNA whatsoever.

In Plants

In plants, it has also been reported that mitochondria can occasionally be inherited from the father, e.g. in bananas. Some Conifers also show paternal inheritance of mitochondria, such as the coast redwood, *Sequoia sempervirens*.

Structure

In humans (and probably in metazoans in general), 100-10,000 separate copies of mtDNA are usually present per cell (egg and sperm cells are exceptions). In mammals, each double-stranded circular mtDNA molecule consists of 15,000-17,000 base pairs. The two strands of mtDNA are differentiated by their nucleotide content with the guanine rich strand referred to as the heavy strand, and the cytosine rich strand referred to as the light strand. The heavy strand encodes 28 genes, and the light strand encodes 9 genes for a total of 37 genes. Of the 37 genes, 13 are for proteins (polypeptides), 22 are for transfer RNA (tRNA) and two are for the small and large subunits of ribosomal RNA (rRNA). This pattern is also seen among most metazoans, although in some cases one or more of the 37 genes is absent and the mtDNA size range is greater. Even greater variation in mtDNA gene content and size exists among fungi and plants, although there appears to be a core subset of genes that are present in all eukaryotes (except for the few that have no mitochondria at all). Some plant species have enormous mtDNAs (as many as 2,500,000 base pairs per mtDNA molecule) but, surprisingly, even those huge mtDNAs contain the same number and kinds of genes as related plants with much smaller mtDNAs.

Genes

Transport Chain

Many of the genes encode the transport chain:

Category	*Genes*
NADH dehydrogenase(complex I)	MT-ND1, MT-ND2, MT-ND3, MT-ND4, MT-ND4L, MT-ND5, MT-ND6
Coenzyme Q - cytochrome c reductase/Cytochrome b(complex III)	MT-CYB
cytochrome c oxidase(complex IV)	MT-CO1, MT-CO2, MT-CO3
ATP synthase	MT-ATP6, MT-ATP8

rRNA

Mitochondrial rRNA is encoded by MT-RNR1 (12S) and MT-RNR2 (16S).

tRNA

The following genes encode tRNA:

Amino Acid	*3-Letter*	*1-Letter*	*MT DNA*
Alanine	Ala	A	MT-TA
Arginine	Arg	R	MT-TR
Asparagine	Asn	N	MT-TN
Aspartic acid	Asp	D	MT-TD
Cysteine	Cys	C	MT-TC

Glutamic acid	Glu	E	MT-TE
Glutamine	Gln	Q	MT-TQ
Glycine	Gly	G	MT-TG
Histidine	His	H	MT-TH
Isoleucine	Ile	I	MT-TI
Leucine	Leu	L	MT-TL1, MT-TL2
Lysine	Lys	K	MT-TK
Methionine	Met	M	MT-TM
Phenylalanine	Phe	F	MT-TF
Proline	Pro	P	MT-TP
Serine	Ser	S	MT-TS1, MT-TS2
Threonine	Thr	T	MT-TT
Tryptophan	Trp	W	MT-TW
Tyrosine	Tyr	Y	MT-TY
Valine	Val	V	MT-TV

Susceptibility

mtDNA is particularly susceptible to reactive oxygen species generated by the respiratory chain due to its close proximity.

Though mtDNA is packaged by proteins and harbors significant DNA repair capacity, these protective functions are less robust than those operating on nuclear DNA and therefore thought to contribute to enhanced susceptibility of mtDNA to oxidative damage.

Genetic Illness

Mutations of mitochondrial DNA can lead to a number of illnesses including exercise intolerance and Kearns-Sayre syndrome (KSS), which causes a person to lose full function of heart, eye, and muscle movements. Some evidence suggests that they might be major contributors to the aging process and age-associated pathologies.

Use in Identification

In humans, mitochondrial DNA spans 16,569 DNA building blocks (base pairs), representing a fraction of the total DNA in cells. Unlike nuclear DNA, which is inherited from both parents and in which genes are rearranged in the process of recombination, there is usually no change in mtDNA from parent to offspring. Although mtDNA also recombines, it does so with copies of itself within the same mitochondrion. Because of this and because the mutation rate of animal mtDNA is higher than that of nuclear DNA, mtDNA is a powerful tool for tracking ancestry through females (matrilineage) and has been used in this role to track the ancestry of many species back hundreds of generations.

Human mtDNA can also be used to help identify individuals. Forensic laboratories occasionally use mtDNA comparison to identify human remains, and especially to identify older unidentified skeletal remains. Although unlike nuclear DNA, mtDNA is not specific to one individual, it can be used in combination with other evidence (anthropological evidence, circumstantial evidence, and the like) to establish identification. mtDNA is also used to exclude possible matches between missing persons and unidentified remains. Many researchers believe that mtDNA is better suited to identification of older skeletal remains than nuclear DNA because the greater number of copies of mtDNA per cell increases the chance of obtaining a useful sample, and because a match with a living relative is possible even if numerous maternal generations separate the two. American outlaw Jesse James's remains were identified using a comparison between mtDNA extracted from his remains and the mtDNA of the son of the female-line great-granddaughter of his sister. Similarly, the remains of Alexandra Feodorovna (Alix of Hesse), last Empress of Russia, and her children were identified by comparison of their mitochondrial DNA with that of Prince Philip, Duke of Edinburgh, whose maternal grandmother was Alexandra's sister Victoria of Hesse. Similarly to identify Emperor Nicholas II remains his mitochondrial DNA was compared with that of James Carnegie, 3rd Duke of Fife, whose maternal great-grandmother Alexandra of Denmark (Queen Alexandra) was sister of Nicholas II mother Dagmar of Denmark (Empress Maria Feodorovna).

The low effective population size and rapid mutation rate (in animals) makes mtDNA useful for assessing genetic relationships of individuals or groups within a species and also for identifying and quantifying the phylogeny (evolutionary relationships) among different species, provided they are not too distantly related. To do this, biologists determine and then compare the mtDNA sequences from different individuals or species. Data from the comparisons is used to construct a network of relationships among the sequences, which provides an estimate of the relationships among the individuals or species from which the mtDNAs were taken. This approach has limits that are imposed by the rate of mtDNA sequence change. In animals, the high mutation rate makes mtDNA most useful for comparisons of individuals within species and for comparisons of species that are closely or moderately-closely related, among which the number of sequence differences can be easily counted. As the species become more distantly related, the number of sequence differences becomes very large; changes begin to accumulate on changes until an accurate count becomes impossible.

History

Mitochondrial DNA was discovered in the 1960s by Margit M. K. Nass and Sylvan Nass by electron microscopy as DNase-sensitive thread inside mitochondria, and by Ellen Haslbrunner, Hans Tuppy and Gottfried Schatz by biochemical assays on highly purified mitochondrial fractions.

National DNA Database

A national DNA database is a government database of DNA profiles which can be used by law enforcement agencies to identify suspects of crimes.

The first government datatabase (NDNAD) was set up by the United Kingdom in April 1995. The second one was set up in New Zealand. France set up the FNAEG in 1998. In the USA, the FBI has organized the CODIS database. Originally intended for sex offenders, they have since been extended to include almost any criminal offender.

In England and Wales, anyone arrested on suspicion of a recordable offence must submit a DNA sample, the profile of which is then stored on the DNA database as a permanent record. In Scotland, the law requires the DNA profiles of most people who are acquitted be removed from the database. In Sweden, only the DNA profiles of criminals who have spent more than two years in prison are stored. In Norway and Germany, court orders are required, and are only available, respectively, for serious offenders and for those convicted of certain offences and who are likely to reoffend. All 50 states in the USA store DNA profiles of violent offenders, and a few also store profiles of suspects. Portugal has plans to introduce a DNA database of its entire population

In Denmark the Danish Newborn Screening Biobank at Statens Serum Institut keeps a blood sample from people born after 1981. The purpose is to test for Phenylketonuria and other diseases . But it is also used for DNA tests to identify diseased and suspected criminals. Parents can request that the blood sample of their newborn is destroyed after the result of test is known.

Scope of Databases

The United States maintains the largest DNA database in the world, with the Combined DNA Index System (CODIS) holding over

5 million records as of 2007. The United Kingdom maintains the National DNA Database (NDNAD), which is of similar size. The size of this database, and its rate of growth, is giving concern to civil liberties and political groups in the UK, where police have wide-ranging powers to take samples and retain them even in the event of acquittal. When a match is made from a national DNA database to link a crime scene to an offender who has provided a DNA sample to a database that link is often referred to as a *cold hit*. A cold hit is of value in referring the police agency to a specific suspect but is of less evidential value than a DNA match made from outside the DNA database..

As of May 2007, 177,870 forensic profiles and 4,582,516 offender profiles have been accumulated, making it the largest DNA database in the world, surpassing the United Kingdom National DNA Database, which consisted of an estimated 3,976,090 profiles as of June 2007. As of the same date, CODIS has produced over 49,400 matches to requests, assisting in more than 50,343 investigations.

The growing public approval of DNA databases has seen the creation and expansion of many states' own DNA databases. California currently maintains the third largest DNA database in the world (naturally, as CODIS contains all states' database information). Political measures such as California Proposition 69 (2004), which increased the scope of the DNA database, have already met with a significant increase in numbers of investigations aided.

In order to decrease the number of irrelevant matches at NDIS, the Convicted Offender Index requires all 13 CODIS STRs to be present for a profile upload. Forensic profiles only require 10 of the STRs to be present for an upload.

DNA Databases and Medicine

The database became the common meeting ground for computer scientists and molecular biologists. This is because the goal of certain projects like the genome project was to construct maps, which were built from information contributed to databases. They enabled an entirely new way of information analysis. Many types of modern molecular biological analysis require computational analysis in parallel. However, the information gained from mapping and sequencing genetic information would very likely have ethical implications for individuals, families and society in general. There is a concern about genetic information being used in ways that affect chances of employment or chance of getting life insurance. Furthermore, secondary applications of personal, genetic information mean that citizens do not know what their genetic information will be used for.

DNA Collection and Human Rights

In a judgement in December 2008, the European Court of Human Rights ruled that two British men should not have had their DNA and fingerprints retained by police saying that retention "could not be regarded as necessary in a democratic society".

The DNA fingerprinting pioneer Professor Sir Alec Jeffreys condemned UK government plans to keep the genetic details of hundreds of thousands of innocent people in England and Wales for up to 12 years. Jeffreys said he was "disappointed" with the proposals, which came after a European court ruled that the current policy breaches people's right to privacy. Jefferys said "It seems to be as about as minimal a response to the European court of human rights judgment as one could conceive. There is a presumption not of innocence but of future guilt here ... which I find very disturbing indeed".

Considerations when Evaluating DNA Evidence

In the early days of the use of genetic fingerprinting as criminal evidence, juries were often swayed by spurious statistical arguments by defence lawyers along these lines: given a match that had a 1 in 5 million probability of occurring by chance, the lawyer would argue that this meant that in a country of say 60 million people there were 12 people who would also match the profile. This was then translated to a 1 in 12 chance of the suspect being the guilty one. This argument is not sound unless the suspect was drawn at random from the population of the country. In fact, a jury should consider how likely it is that an individual matching the genetic profile would also have been a suspect in the case for other reasons. Another spurious statistical argument is based on the false assumption that a 1 in 5 million probability of a match automatically translates into a 1 in 5 million probability of innocence and is known as the prosecutor's fallacy.

When using RFLP, the theoretical risk of a coincidental match is 1 in 100 billion (100,000,000,000), although the practical risk is actually 1 in 1000 because monozygotic twins are 0.2% of the human population. Moreover, the rate of laboratory error is almost certainly higher than this, and often actual laboratory procedures do not reflect the theory under which the coincidence probabilities were computed. For example, the coincidence probabilities may be calculated based on the probabilities that markers in two samples have bands in *precisely* the same location, but a laboratory worker may conclude that similar—but not precisely identical—band patterns result from identical genetic samples with some imperfection in the agarose gel. However, in this case, the laboratory worker increases the coincidence risk by expanding the criteria for declaring a match. Recent studies have quoted relatively high error rates which may be cause for concern. In the early days of genetic fingerprinting, the necessary population data to accurately compute a match probability was sometimes unavailable. Between 1992 and 1996, arbitrary low ceilings were controversially put on match probabilities used in RFLP analysis rather than the higher theoretically computed ones. Today, RFLP has become widely disused due to the advent of more discriminating, sensitive and easier technologies.

STRs do not suffer from such subjectivity and provide similar power of discrimination (1 in 10^13 for unrelated individuals if using a full SGM+ profile) It should be noted that figures of this magnitude are not considered to be statistically supportable by scientists in the UK, for unrelated individuals with full matching DNA profiles a match probability of 1 in a billion is considered statistically supportable (Since 1998 the DNA profiling system supported by The National DNA Database in the UK is the SGM+ DNA profiling system which includes 10 STR regions and a sex indicating test. However, with any DNA technique, the cautious juror should not convict on genetic fingerprint evidence alone if other factors raise doubt. Contamination with other evidence (secondary transfer) is a key source of incorrect DNA profiles and raising doubts as to whether a sample has been adulterated is a favorite defence technique. More rarely, chimerism is one such instance where the lack of a genetic match may unfairly exclude a suspect.

Evidence of Genetic Relationship

It's also possible to use DNA profiling as evidence of genetic relationship, but testing that shows no relationship isn't absolutely certain. While almost all individuals have a single and distinct set of genes, rare individuals, known as "chimeras", have at least two different sets of genes. There have been several cases of DNA profiling that falsely "proved" that a mother was unrelated to her children.

Fake DNA Evidence

The value of DNA evidence has to be seen in light of recent cases where criminals planted fake DNA samples at crime scenes. In one case, a criminal even planted fake DNA evidence in his own body: Dr.

John Schneeberger raped one of his sedated patients in 1992 and left semen on her underwear. Police drew what they believed to be Schneeberger's blood and compared its DNA against the crime scene semen DNA on three occasions, never showing a match. It turned out that he had surgically inserted a Penrose drain into his arm and filled it with foreign blood and anticoagulants.

In a study conducted by the life science company Nucleix and published in the journal Forensic Science International, scientists found that an In vitro synthesized sample of DNA matching any desired genetic profile can be constructed using standard molecular biology techniques without obtaining any actual tissue from that person.

In the case of the Phantom of Heilbronn, police detectives found DNA traces from the same woman on various crime scenes in Austria, Germany and France - among them murders, burglaries and robberies. Only after the DNA of the "woman" matched the DNA sampled from the burned body of a *male* asylum seeker in France, detectives began to have serious doubts about the DNA evidence. In that case, DNA traces were already present on the cotton swabs used to collect the samples at the crime scene, and the swabs had all been produced at the same factory in Austria. The company's product specification said that the swabs were guaranteed to be sterile, but not DNA-free.

Familial Searching

Familial searching is the use of family members' DNA to identify a closely related suspect in jurisdictions where large DNA databases exist, but no exact match has been found. The first successful use of the practice was in a UK case where a man was convicted of manslaughter when he threw a brick stained with his own blood into a moving car. Police could not get an exact match to the UK's DNA database because the man had no criminal convictions, but police implicated him using a close relative's DNA. The technique was used to catch a Los Angeles serial killer known as the "Grim Sleeper" in 2010.

Surreptitious DNA Collecting

Police forces may collect DNA samples without the suspects' knowledge, and use it as evidence. Legality of this mode of proceeding has been questioned in Australia.

In the United States, it has been accepted, courts often claiming that there was no expectation of privacy, citing California v. Greenwood

(1985), during which the Supreme Court held that the Fourth Amendment does not prohibit the warrantless search and seizure of garbage left for collection outside the curtilage of a home. Critics of this practice underline the fact that this analogy ignores that "most people have no idea that they risk surrendering their genetic identity to the police by, for instance, failing to destroy a used coffee cup. Moreover, even if they do realize it, there is no way to avoid abandoning one's DNA in public."

In the UK, the Human Tissue Act 2004 prohibited private individuals from covertly collecting biological samples (hair, fingernails, etc.) for DNA analysis, but excluded medical and criminal investigations from the offense.

England and Wales

Evidence from an expert who has compared DNA samples must be accompanied by evidence as to the sources of the samples and the procedures for obtaining the DNA profiles. The judge must ensure that the jury must understand the significance of DNA matches and mismatches in the profiles.

The judge must also ensure that the jury does not confuse the 'match probability' (the probability that a person that is chosen at random has a matching DNA profile to the sample from the scene) with the 'likelihood ratio' (the probability that a person with matching DNA committed the crime). In *R v. Doheny* Phillips LJ gave this example of a summing up, which should be carefully tailored to the particular facts in each case:

Members of the Jury, if you accept the scientific evidence called by the Crown, this indicates that there are probably only four or five white males in the United Kingdom from whom that semen stain could have come.

The Defendant is one of them. If that is the position, the decision you have to reach, on all the evidence, is whether you are sure that it was the Defendant who left that stain or whether it is possible that it was one of that other small group of men who share the same DNA characteristics.

Juries should weigh up conflicting and corroborative evidence, using their own common sense and not by using mathematical formulae, such as Bayes' theorem, so as to avoid "confusion, misunderstanding and misjudgment".

Presentation and Evaluation of Evidence of Partial or Incomplete DNA Profiles

In *R v Bates*, Moore-Bick LJ said:

> *"We can see no reason why partial profile DNA evidence should not be admissible provided that the jury are made aware of its inherent limitations and are given a sufficient explanation to enable them to evaluate it. There may be cases where the match probability in relation to all the samples tested is so great that the judge would consider its probative value to be minimal and decide to exclude the evidence in the exercise of his discretion, but this gives rise to no new question of principle and can be left for decision on a case by case basis. However, the fact that there exists in the case of all partial profile evidence the possibility that a "missing" allele might exculpate the accused altogether does not provide sufficient grounds for rejecting such evidence. In many there is a possibility (at least in theory) that evidence exists which would assist the accused and perhaps even exculpate him altogether, but that does not provide grounds for excluding relevant evidence that is available and otherwise admissible, though it does make it important to ensure that the jury are given sufficient information to enable them to evaluate that evidence properly".*

DNA Testing in the US

There are state laws on DNA profiling in all 50 states of the United States. Detailed information on database laws in each state can be found at the National Conference of State Legislatures website.

Development of Artificial DNA

In August 2009, scientists in Israel stunned the forensic sciences and raised serious questions concerning the use of DNA by law enforcement as the ultimate method of identification. In a paper published in the journal *Forensic Science International: Genetics*, the Israeli researchers demonstrated that it is possible to manufacture DNA in a laboratory, and thus falsify DNA evidence.

The scientists fabricated saliva and blood samples, which originally contained DNA from a person other than the ostensible donor of the blood and saliva.

The researchers also showed that, using a DNA database, it is possible to take information from a profile and manufacture DNA to match it, and that this can be done without access to any actual DNA from the person whose DNA they are duplicating. The synthetic DNA oligos required for the procedure are common in molecular laboratories.

Dr. Daniel Frumkin, lead author on the paper, was quoted in *The New York Times* as saying, "You can just engineer a crime scene... any biology undergraduate could perform this." Dr. Frumkin perfected a test that can forensically differentiate real DNA samples from fake ones. His test detects epigenetic modifications, in particular, DNA methylation.

Seventy percent of the DNA in any human genome is methylated, meaning it contains methyl group modifications within a CpG dinucleotide context. Methylation at the promoter region is associated with gene silencing. The synthetic DNA lacks this epigenetic modification, which allows the test to distinguish manufactured DNA from original, genuine, DNA.

It is unknown how many, if any, police departments currently use the test, which appears to be a serious issue in light of Frumkin's claim that the DNA manufacturing procedure is within the grasp of any undergraduate biology student. No police lab has publicly announced that it is using the new test to verify DNA results, while FSI Genetics says that any forensic laboratory doing DNA identification should adopt this test to authenticate its results as "real" DNA.

Cases

- In the 1950s, Anna Anderson claimed that she was Grand Duchess Anastasia Nikolaevna of Russia; in the 1980s after her death, samples of her tissue that had been stored at a Charlottesville, Virginia hospital following a medical procedure were tested using DNA fingerprinting and showed that she bore no relation to the Romanovs.
- In 1986, Richard Buckland was exonerated despite having admitted to the rape and murder of a teenager near Leicester, the city where DNA profiling was first discovered. This was the first use of DNA finger printing in a criminal investigation.
- In 1987, in the same case as Buckland, British baker Colin Pitchfork was the first criminal caught and convicted using DNA fingerprinting.
- In 1987, genetic fingerprinting was used in criminal court for the first time in the trial of a man accused of unlawful

intercourse with a mentally handicapped 14-year-old female who gave birth to his baby.

- In 1987, Florida rapist Tommy Lee Andrews was the first person in the United States to be convicted as a result of DNA evidence, for raping a woman during a burglary; he was convicted on 6 November 1987 and sentenced to 22 years in prison.
- In 1988, Timothy Spencer was the first man in Virginia to be sentenced to death through DNA testing, for several rape and murder charges; he was dubbed "The South Side Strangler" because he killed victims on the southside of Richmond, Virginia. He was later charged with rape and 1st degree murder and was sentenced to death. He was executed on April 27, 1994. David Vasquez, initially convicted of one of Spencer's crimes, became the first man in America exonerated based on DNA evidence.
- In 1989, Chicago man Gary Dotson was the first person whose conviction was overturned using DNA evidence.
- In 1991, Allan Legere was the first Canadian to be convicted as a result of DNA evidence, for four murders he had committed while an escaped prisoner in 1989. During his trial, his defence argued that the relatively shallow gene pool of the region could lead to false positives.
- In 1992, DNA evidence was used to prove that Nazi doctor Josef Mengele was buried in Brazil under the name Wolfgang Gerhard.
- In 1993, Kirk Bloodsworth was the first person to have been convicted of murder and sentenced to death, whose conviction was overturned using DNA evidence.
- The 1993 rape and murder of Mia Zapata, lead singer for the Seattle punk band The Gits was unsolved 9 years after the murder. A database search in 2001 failed, but the killer's DNA was collected when he was arrested in Florida for burglary and domestic abuse in 2002.
- The science was made famous in the United States in 1994 when prosecutors heavily relied on — and through expert witnesses exhaustively presented and explained — DNA evidence allegedly linking O.J. Simpson to a double murder. The case also brought to light the laboratory difficulties and handling procedure mishaps which can cause such evidence to be significantly doubted.

- In 1994, Royal Canadian Mounted Police (RCMP) detectives successfully tested hairs from a cat known as Snowball, and used the test to link a man to the murder of his wife, thus marking for the first time in forensic history the use of non-human DNA to identify a criminal.
- In 1998, Dr. Richard J. Schmidt was convicted of attempted second-degree murder when it was shown that there was a link between the viral DNA of the human immunodeficiency virus (HIV) he had been accused of injecting in his girlfriend and viral DNA from one of his patients with full-blown AIDS. This was the first time viral DNA fingerprinting had been used as evidence in a criminal trial.
- In 1999, Raymond Easton a disabled man from Swindon, England was arrested and detained for 7 hours in connection with a burglary due to an inaccurrate DNA match. His DNA had been retained on file after an unrelated domestic incident some time previously.
- In May 2000 Gordon Graham murdered Paul Gault at his home in Lisburn, Northern Ireland. Graham was convicted of the murder when his DNA was found on a sports bag left in the house as part of an elaborate ploy to suggest the murder occurred after a burglary had gone wrong. Graham was having an affair with the victims wife at the time of the murder. It was the first time Low Copy Number DNA was used in Northern Ireland.
- In 2001, Wayne Butler was convicted for the murder of Celia Douty. It was the first murder in Australia to be solved using DNA profiling.
- In 2002, DNA testing was used to exonerate Douglas Echols, a man who was wrongfully convicted in a 1986 rape case. Echols was the 114th person to be exonerated through post-conviction DNA testing.
- In August 2002, Annalisa Vincenzi was shot dead in Tuscany. Some time later, Bartender Peter Hamkin, 23, was arrested in Merseyside in March 2003 on an extradition warrant heard at Bow Street Magistrates' Court in London to establish whether he should be taken to Italy to face a murder charge. DNA "proved" he shot her, but he was cleared on other evidence.
- In 2003, Welshman Jeffrey Gafoor was convicted of the 1988 murder of Lynette White, when crime scene evidence collected

12 years earlier was re-examined using STR techniques, resulting in a match with his nephew. This may be the first known example of the DNA of an innocent yet related individual being used to identify the actual criminal, via "familial searching".

- In June 2003, because of new DNA evidence, Dennis Halstead, John Kogut and John Restivo won a re-trial on their murder conviction. The three men had already served eighteen years of their thirty-plus-year sentences.
- The trial of Robert Pickton is notable in that DNA evidence is being used primarily to identify the *victims*, and in many cases to prove their existence.
- In March 2003, Josiah Sutton was released from prison after serving four years of a twelve-year sentence for a sexual assault charge. Questionable DNA samples taken from Sutton were retested in the wake of the Houston Police Department's crime lab scandal of mishandling DNA evidence.
- In 2004, DNA testing shed new light into the mysterious 1912 disappearance of Bobby Dunbar, a four-year-old boy who vanished during a fishing trip. He was allegedly found alive eight months later in the custody of William Cantwell Walters, but another woman claimed that the boy was her son, Bruce Anderson, whom she had entrusted in Walters' custody. The courts disbelieved her claim and convicted Walters for the kidnapping.

  The boy was raised and known as Bobby Dunbar throughout the rest of his life. However, DNA tests on Dunbar's son and nephew revealed the two were not related, thus establishing that the boy found in 1912 was not Bobby Dunbar, whose real fate remains unknown.
- In 2005, Gary Leiterman was convicted of the 1969 murder of Jane Mixer, a law student at the University of Michigan, after DNA found on Mixer's pantyhose was matched to Leiterman. DNA in a drop of blood on Mixer's hand was matched to John Ruelas, who was only four years old in 1969 and was never successfully connected to the case in any other way. Leiterman's defence unsuccessfully argued that the unexplained match of the blood spot to Ruelas pointed to cross-contamination and raised doubts about the reliability of the lab's identification of Leiterman.

- In December 2005, Evan Simmons was proven innocent of a 1981 attack on an Atlanta woman after serving twenty-four years in prison. Mr Clark is the 164th person in the United States and the fifth in Georgia to be freed using post-conviction DNA testing.
- In March 2009, Sean Hodgson who spent 27 years in jail, convicted of killing Teresa De Simone, 22, in her car in Southampton 30 years ago was quashed by senior judges. Tests prove DNA from the scene was not his. British police have now reopened the case.

Bioinformatics

Bioinformatics is the application of statistics and computer science to the field of molecular biology.

The term *bioinformatics* was coined by Paulien Hogeweg and Ben Hesper in 1978 for the study of informatic processes in biotic systems. Its primary use since at least the late 1980s has been in genomics and genetics, particularly in those areas of genomics involving large-scale DNA sequencing.

Bioinformatics now entails the creation and advancement of databases, algorithms, computational and statistical techniques and theory to solve formal and practical problems arising from the management and analysis of biological data.

Over the past few decades rapid developments in genomic and other molecular research technologies and developments in information technologies have combined to produce a tremendous amount of information related to molecular biology. It is the name given to these mathematical and computing approaches used to glean understanding of biological processes.

Common activities in bioinformatics include mapping and analyzing DNA and protein sequences, aligning different DNA and protein sequences to compare them and creating and viewing 3-D models of protein structures.

The primary goal of bioinformatics is to increase the understanding of biological processes. What sets it apart from other approaches, however, is its focus on developing and applying computationally intensive techniques (e.g., pattern recognition, data mining, machine learning algorithms, and visualization) to achieve this goal. Major research efforts in the field include sequence alignment, gene finding, genome assembly, drug design, drug discovery, protein structure alignment, protein structure prediction, prediction of gene expression and protein-protein interactions, genome-wide association studies and the modelling of evolution.

Bioinformatics was applied in the creation and maintenance of a database to store biological information at the beginning of the "genomic revolution", such as nucleotide and amino acid sequences. Development of this type of database involved not only design issues but the development of complex interfaces whereby researchers could both access existing data as well as submit new or revised data.

In order to study how normal cellular activities are altered in different disease states, the biological data must be combined to form a comprehensive picture of these activities. Therefore, the field of bioinformatics has evolved such that the most pressing task now involves the analysis and interpretation of various types of data, including nucleotide and amino acid sequences, protein domains, and protein structures. The actual process of analyzing and interpreting data is referred to as computational biology. Important sub-disciplines within bioinformatics and computational biology include:

- the development and implementation of tools that enable efficient access to, and use and management of, various types of information.
- the development of new algorithms (mathematical formulas) and statistics with which to assess relationships among members of large data sets, such as methods to locate a gene within a sequence, predict protein structure and/or function, and cluster protein sequences into families of related sequences.

There are two fundamental ways of modelling a Biological system (e.g. living cell) both coming under Bioinformatic approaches.

- Static
  - o Sequences - Proteins, Nucleic acids and Peptides
  - o Structures - Proteins, Nucleic acids, Ligands (including metabolites and drugs) and Peptides
  - o Interaction data among the above entities including microarray data and Networks of proteins, metabolites
- Dynamic
  - o Systems Biology comes under this category including reaction fluxes and variable concentrations of metabolites

- o Multi-Agent Based modelling approaches capturing cellular events such as signalling, transcription and reaction dynamics.

A broad sub-category under bioinformatics is structural bioinformatics.

Major Research Areas

Sequence Analysis

Since the Phage F-X174 was sequenced in 1977, the DNA sequences of thousands of organisms have been decoded and stored in databases. This sequence information is analysed to determine genes that encode polypeptides (proteins), RNA genes, regulatory sequences, structural motifs, and repetitive sequences. A comparison of genes within a species or between different species can show similarities between protein functions, or relations between species (the use of molecular systematics to construct phylogenetic trees). With the growing amount of data, it long ago became impractical to analyse DNA sequences manually. Today, computer programs such as BLAST are used daily to search sequences from more than 260 000 organisms, containing over 190 billion nucleotides. These programs can compensate for mutations (exchanged, deleted or inserted bases) in the DNA sequence, in order to identify sequences that are related, but not identical. A variant of this sequence alignment is used in the sequencing process itself. The so-called shotgun sequencing technique (which was used, for example, by The Institute for Genomic Research to sequence the first bacterial genome, *Haemophilus influenzae*) does not produce entire chromosomes, but instead generates the sequences of many thousands of small DNA fragments (ranging from 35 to 900 nucleotides long, depending on the sequencing technology).

The ends of these fragments overlap and, when aligned properly by a genome assembly program, can be used to reconstruct the complete genome. Shotgun sequencing yields sequence data quickly, but the task of assembling the fragments can be quite complicated for larger genomes. For a genome as large as the human genome, it may take many days of CPU time on large-memory, multiprocessor computers to assemble the fragments, and the resulting assembly will usually contain numerous gaps that have to be filled in later. Shotgun sequencing is the method of choice for virtually all genomes sequenced today, and genome assembly algorithms are a critical area of bioinformatics research.

Another aspect of bioinformatics in sequence analysis is annotation, which involves computational gene finding to search for protein-coding genes, RNA genes, and other functional sequences within a genome. Not all of the nucleotides within a genome are part of genes. Within the genome of higher organisms, large parts of the DNA do not serve any obvious purpose. This so-called junk DNA may, however, contain unrecognized functional elements. Bioinformatics helps to bridge the gap between genome and proteome projects — for example, in the use of DNA sequences for protein identification.

Gene Prediction

Gene finding typically refers to the area of computational biology that is concerned with algorithmically identifying stretches of sequence, usually genomic DNA, that are biologically functional. This especially includes protein-coding genes, but may also include other functional elements such as RNA genes and regulatory regions. Gene finding is one of the first and most important steps in understanding the genome of a species once it has been sequenced.

In its earliest days, "gene finding" was based on painstaking experimentation on living cells and organisms. Statistical analysis of the rates of homologous recombination of several different genes could determine their order on a certain chromosome, and information from many such experiments could be combined to create a genetic map specifying the rough location of known genes relative to each other. Today, with comprehensive genome sequence and powerful computational resources at the disposal of the research community, gene finding has been redefined as a largely computational problem. Determining that a sequence *is functional* should be distinguished from determining *the function* of the gene or its product. The latter still demands *in vivo* experimentation through gene knockout and other assays, although frontiers of bioinformatics research are making it increasingly possible to predict the function of a gene based on its sequence alone.

Extrinsic Approaches

In extrinsic (or evidence-based) gene finding systems, the target genome is searched for sequences that are similar to extrinsic evidence in the form of the known sequence of a messenger RNA (mRNA) or protein product. Given an mRNA sequence, it is trivial to derive a unique genomic DNA sequence from which it had to have been transcribed. Given a protein sequence, a family of possible coding

DNA sequences can be derived by reverse translation of the genetic code. Once candidate DNA sequences have been determined, it is a relatively straightforward algorithmic problem to efficiently search a target genome for matches, complete or partial, and exact or inexact. BLAST is a widely used system designed for this purpose.

A high degree of similarity to a known messenger RNA or protein product is strong evidence that a region of a target genome is a protein-coding gene. However, to apply this approach systemically requires extensive sequencing of mRNA and protein products. Not only is this expensive, but in complex organisms, only a subset of all genes in the organism's genome are expressed at any given time, meaning that extrinsic evidence for many genes is not readily accessible in any single cell culture. Thus, in order to collect extrinsic evidence for most or all of the genes in a complex organism, many hundreds or thousands of different cell types must be studied, which itself presents further difficulties. For example, some human genes may be expressed only during development as an embryo or fetus , which might be difficult to study for ethical reasons.

Despite these difficulties, extensive transcript and protein sequence databases have been generated for human as well as other important model organisms in biology, such as mice and yeast. For example, the RefSeq database contains transcript and protein sequence from many different species, and the Ensembl system comprehensively maps this evidence to human and several other genomes. It is, however, likely that these databases are both incomplete and contain small but significant amounts of erroneous data..

Ab Initio Approaches

Because of the inherent expense and difficulty in obtaining extrinsic evidence for many genes, it is also necessary to resort to *Ab initio* gene finding, in which genomic DNA sequence alone is systematically searched for certain tell-tale signs of protein-coding genes. These signs can be broadly categorized as either *signals*, specific sequences that indicate the presence of a gene nearby, or *content*, statistical properties of protein-coding sequence itself. *Ab initio* gene finding might be more accurately characterized as gene *prediction*, since extrinsic evidence is generally required to conclusively establish that a putative gene is functional.

In the genomes of prokaryotes, genes have specific and relatively well-understood promoter sequences (signals), such as the Pribnow box and transcription factor binding sites, which are easy to systematically identify. Also, the sequence coding for a protein occurs as one contiguous open reading frame (ORF), which is typically many hundred or thousands of base pairs long. The statistics of stop codons are such that even finding an open reading frame of this length is a fairly informative sign. (Since 3 of the 64 possible codons in the genetic code are stop codons, one would expect a stop codon approximately every 20-25 codons, or 60-75 base pairs, in a random sequence.) Furthermore, protein-coding DNA has certain periodicities and other statistical properties that are easy to detect in sequence of this length. These characteristics make prokaryotic gene finding relatively straightforward, and well-designed systems are able to achieve high levels of accuracy.

Ab initio gene finding in eukaryotes, especially complex organisms like humans, is considerably more challenging for several reasons. First, the promoter and other regulatory signals in these genomes are more complex and less well-understood than in prokaryotes, making them more difficult to reliably recognize. Two classic examples of signals identified by eukaryotic gene finders are CpG islands and binding sites for a poly(A) tail.

Second, splicing mechanisms employed by eukaryotic cells mean that a particular protein-coding sequence in the genome is divided into several parts (exons), separated by non-coding sequences (introns). (Splice sites are themselves another signal that eukaryotic gene finders are often designed to identify.) A typical protein-coding gene in humans might be divided into a dozen exons, each less than two hundred base pairs in length, and some as short as twenty to thirty. It is therefore much more difficult to detect periodicities and other known content properties of protein-coding DNA in eukaryotes.

Advanced gene finders for both prokaryotic and eukaryotic genomes typically use complex probabilistic models, such as hidden Markov models, in order to combine information from a variety of different signal and content measurements. The GLIMMER system is a widely used and highly accurate gene finder for prokaryotes. GeneMark is another popular approach. Eukaryotic *ab initio* gene finders, by comparison, have achieved only limited success; notable examples are the GENSCAN and geneid programs. The SNAP gene finder is HMM-based like Genscan and attempts to be more adaptable to different organisms, addressing problems related to using a gene finder on a genome sequence that it was not trained against.A few recent approaches like mSplicer, CONTRAST, or mGene also use machine learning techniques like support vector machines for successful gene prediction. They build a discriminative model using hidden Markov support vector machines or conditional random fields to learn an accurate gene prediction scoring function.

Other Signals

Among the derived signals used for prediction are statistics resulting from the sub-sequence statistics like k-mer statistics, Fourier transform of a pseudo-number-coded DNA, Z-curve parameters and certain run features.

It has been suggested that signals other than those directly detectable in sequences may improve gene prediction. For example, the role of secondary structure in the identification of regulatory motifs has been reported. In addition, it has been suggested that RNA secondary structure prediction helps splice site prediction.

Comparative Genomics Approaches

As the entire genomes of many different species are sequenced, a promising direction in current research on gene finding is a comparative genomics approach. This is based on the principle that the forces of natural selection cause genes and other functional elements to undergo mutation at a slower rate than the rest of the genome, since mutations in functional elements are more likely to negatively impact the organism than mutations elsewhere. Genes can thus be detected by comparing the genomes of related species to detect this evolutionary pressure for conservation. This approach was first applied to the mouse and human genomes, using programs such as SLAM, SGP and Twinscan/N-SCAN.

Comparative gene finding can also be used to project high quality annotations from one genome to another. Notable examples include Projector, GeneWise and GeneMapper. Such techniques now play a central role in the annotation of all genomes.

Computational Evolutionary Biology

Evolutionary biology is the study of the origin and descent of species, as well as their change over time. Informatics has assisted evolutionary biologists in several key ways; it has enabled researchers to:

- trace the evolution of a large number of organisms by measuring changes in their DNA, rather than through physical taxonomy or physiological observations alone,
- more recently, compare entire genomes, which permits the study of more complex evolutionary events, such as gene

duplication, horizontal gene transfer, and the prediction of factors important in bacterial speciation,

- build complex computational models of populations to predict the outcome of the system over time
- track and share information on an increasingly large number of species and organisms.

Future work endeavours to reconstruct the now more complex tree of life. The area of research within computer science that uses genetic algorithms is sometimes confused with computational evolutionary biology, but the two areas are not necessarily related.

Analysis of Gene Expression

The expression of many genes can be determined by measuring mRNA levels with multiple techniques including microarrays, expressed cDNA sequence tag (EST) sequencing, serial analysis of gene expression (SAGE) tag sequencing, massively parallel signature sequencing (MPSS), or various applications of multiplexed in-situ hybridization. All of these techniques are extremely noise-prone and/or subject to bias in the biological measurement, and a major research area in computational biology involves developing statistical tools to separate signal from noise in high-throughput gene expression studies. Such studies are often used to determine the genes implicated in a disorder: one might compare microarray data from cancerous epithelial cells to data from non-cancerous cells to determine the transcripts that are up-regulated and down-regulated in a particular population of cancer cells.

Analysis of Regulation

Regulation is the complex orchestration of events starting with an extracellular signal such as a hormone and leading to an increase or decrease in the activity of one or more proteins. Bioinformatics techniques have been applied to explore various steps in this process. For example, promoter analysis involves the identification and study of sequence motifs in the DNA surrounding the coding region of a gene. These motifs influence the extent to which that region is transcribed into mRNA. Expression data can be used to infer gene regulation: one might compare microarray data from a wide variety of states of an organism to form hypotheses about the genes involved in each state. In a single-cell organism, one might compare stages of the cell cycle, along with various stress conditions (heat shock, starvation, etc.). One can then apply clustering algorithms to that expression data to determine which genes are co-expressed. For example, the upstream regions (promoters) of co-expressed genes can be searched for over-represented regulatory elements.

Analysis of Protein Expression

Protein microarrays and high throughput (HT) mass spectrometry (MS) can provide a snapshot of the proteins present in a biological sample. Bioinformatics is very much involved in making sense of protein microarray and HT MS data; the former approach faces similar problems as with microarrays targeted at mRNA, the latter involves the problem of matching large amounts of mass data against predicted masses from protein sequence databases, and the complicated statistical analysis of samples where multiple, but incomplete peptides from each protein are detected.

Analysis of Mutations in Cancer

In cancer, the genomes of affected cells are rearranged in complex or even unpredictable ways. Massive sequencing efforts are used to identify previously unknown point mutations in a variety of genes in cancer. Bioinformaticians continue to produce specialized automated systems to manage the sheer volume of sequence data produced, and they create new algorithms and software to compare the sequencing results to the growing collection of human genome sequences and germline polymorphisms. New physical detection technologies are employed, such as oligonucleotide microarrays to identify chromosomal gains and losses (called comparative genomic hybridization), and single-nucleotide polymorphism arrays to detect known *point mutations.* These detection methods simultaneously measure several hundred thousand sites throughout the genome, and when used in high-throughput to measure thousands of samples, generate terabytes of data per experiment. Again the massive amounts and new types of data generate new opportunities for bioinformaticians. The data is often found to contain considerable variability, or noise, and thus Hidden Markov model and change-point analysis methods are being developed to infer real copy number changes.

Another type of data that requires novel informatics development is the analysis of lesions found to be recurrent among many tumours.

Comparative Genomics

Comparative genomics is the study of the relationship of genome structure and function across different biological species or strains. Comparative genomics is an attempt to take advantage of the information provided by the signatures of selection to understand the function and evolutionary processes that act on genomes. While it is still a young field, it holds great promise to yield insights into many aspects of the evolution of modern species. The sheer amount of information contained in modern genomes (3.2 gigabases in the case of humans) necessitates that the methods of comparative genomics are automated. Gene finding is an important application of comparative genomics, as is discovery of new, non-coding functional elements of the genome.

Comparative genomics exploits both similarities and differences in the proteins, RNA, and regulatory regions of different organisms to infer how selection has acted upon these elements. Those elements that are responsible for similarities between different species should be conserved through time (stabilizing selection), while those elements responsible for differences among species should be divergent (positive selection). Finally, those elements that are unimportant to the evolutionary success of the organism will be unconserved (selection is neutral).

One of the important goals of the field is the identification of the mechanisms of eukaryotic genome evolution. It is however often complicated by the multiplicity of events that have taken place throughout the history of individual lineages, leaving only distorted and superimposed traces in the genome of each living organism. For this reason comparative genomics studies of small model organisms (for example yeast) are of great importance to advance our understanding of general mechanisms of evolution.

Having come a long way from its initial use of finding functional proteins, comparative genomics is now concentrating on finding regulatory regions and siRNA molecules. Recently, it has been discovered that distantly related species often share long conserved stretches of DNA that do not appear to code for any protein . One such ultra-conserved region, that was stable from chicken to chimp has undergone a sudden burst of change in the human lineage, and is found to be active in the developing brain of the human embryo.

Computational approaches to genome comparison have recently become a common research topic in computer science. A public collection of case studies and demonstrations is growing, ranging from whole genome comparisons to gene expression analysis. This has increased the introduction of different ideas, including concepts from systems and control, information theory, strings analysis and data mining. It is anticipated that computational approaches will become and remain a standard topic for research and teaching, while multiple courses will begin training students to be fluent in both topics.

Modelling Biological Systems

Modelling biological systems is a significant task of systems biology and mathematical biology. Computational systems biology aims to develop and use efficient algorithms, data structures, visualization and communication tools to orchestrate the integration of large quantities of biological data with the goal of computer modelling. It involves the use of computer simulations of biological systems, like cellular subsystems (such as the networks of metabolites and enzymes which comprise metabolism, signal transduction pathways and gene regulatory networks) to both analyse and visualize the complex connections of these cellular processes.

It is also directly associated with bioinformatics and computational biology. Artificial life or virtual evolution attempts to understand evolutionary processes via the computer simulation of simple (artificial) life forms.

Overview

It is understood that an unexpected emergent property of a complex system is a result of the interplay of the cause-and-effect among simpler, integrated parts. Biological systems manifest many important examples of emergent properties in the complex interplay of components. Traditional study of biological systems requires reductive methods in which quantities of data are gathered by category, such as concentration over time in response to a certain stimulus. Computers are critical to analysis and modelling of these data. The goal is to create accurate real-time models of a system's response to environmental and internal stimuli, such as a model of a cancer cell in order to find weaknesses in its signalling pathways, or modelling of ion channel mutations to see effects on cardiomyocytes and in turn, the function of a beating heart.

A monograph on this topic summarizes an extensive amount of published research in this area up to 1987, including subsections in the following areas: computer modelling in biology and medicine, arterial system models, neuron models, biochemical and oscillation networks, quantum automata, quantum computers in molecular biology and genetics, cancer modelling, neural nets, genetic networks, abstract relational biology, metabolic-replication systems, category theory applications in biology and medicine, automata theory, cellular automata, tessallation models and complete self-reproduction, chaotic systems in organisms, relational biology and organismic theories. This published report also includes 390 references to peer-reviewed articles by a large number of authors.

Standards

By far the most widely accepted standard format for storing and exchanging models in the field is the Systems Biology Markup Language (SBML) The SBML.org website includes a guide to many important software packages used in computational systems biology. Other markup languages with different emphases include BioPAX and CellML.

Particular Tasks

Cellular Model

Creating a cellular model has been a particularly challenging task of systems biology and mathematical biology. It involves developing efficient algorithms, data structures, visualization and communication tools to orchestrate the integration of large quantities of biological data with the goal of computer modelling.

It is also directly associated with bioinformatics, computational biology and Artificial life. It involves the use of computer simulations of the many cellular subsystems such as the networks of metabolites and enzymes which comprise metabolism, signal transduction pathways and gene regulatory networks to both analyse and visualize the complex connections of these cellular processes.

The complex network of biochemical reaction/transport processes and their spatial organization make the development of a predictive model of a living cell a grand challenge for the 21st century.

Overview

The eukaryotic cell cycle is very complex and is one of the most studied topics, since its misregulation leads to cancers. It is possibly a good example of a mathematical model as it deals with simple calculus but gives valid results. Two research groups have produced several models of the cell cycle simulating several organisms. They have recently produced a generic eukaryotic cell cycle model which can represent a particular eukaryote depending on the values of the parameters, demonstrating that the idiosyncrasies of the individual cell cycles are due to different protein concentrations and affinities, while the underlying mechanisms are conserved (Csikasz-Nagy et al., 2006). By means of a system of ordinary differential equations these models show the change in time (dynamical system) of the protein inside a single typical cell; this type of model is called a deterministic process (whereas a model describing a statistical distribution of protein concentrations in a population of cells is called a stochastic process).

To obtain these equations an iterative series of steps must be done: first the several models and observations are combined to form a consensus diagram and the appropriate kinetic laws are chosen to write the differential equations, such as rate kinetics for stoichiometric reactions, Michaelis-Menten kinetics for enzyme substrate reactions and Goldbeter–Koshland kinetics for ultrasensitive transcription factors, afterwards the parameters of the equations (rate constants, enzyme efficiency coefficients and Michealis constants) must be fitted to match observations; when they cannot be fitted the kinetic equation is revised and when that is not possible the wiring diagram is modified. The parameters are fitted and validated using observations of both wild type and mutants, such as protein half-life and cell size.

In order to fit the parameters the differential equations need to be studied. This can be done either by simulation or by analysis.

In a simulation, given a starting vector (list of the values of the variables), the progression of the system is calculated by solving the equations at each time-frame in small increments.

In analysis, the proprieties of the equations are used to investigate the Behaviour of the system depending of the values of the parameters and variables. A system of differential equations can be represented as a vector field, where each vector described the change (in concentration of two or more protein) determining where and how fast the trajectory (simulation) is heading. Vector fields can have several special points: a stable point, called a sink, that attracts in all directions (forcing the concentrations to be at a certain value), an unstable point, either a source or a saddle point which repels (forcing the concentrations to change away from a certain value), and a limit cycle, a closed trajectory towards which several trajectories spiral towards (making the concentrations oscillate).

A better representation which can handle the large number of variables and parameters is called a bifurcation diagram (bifurcation theory): the presence of these special steady-state points at certain values of a parameter (e.g. mass) is represented by a point and once the parameter passes a certain value, a qualitative change occurs, called a bifurcation, in which the nature of the space changes, with profound consequences for the protein concentrations: the cell cycle has phases (partially corresponding to G1 and G2) in which mass, via a stable point, controls cyclin levels, and phases (S and M phases) in which the concentrations change independently, but once the phase has changed at a bifurcation event (cell cycle checkpoint), the system cannot go back to the previous levels since at the current mass the vector field is profoundly different and the mass cannot be reversed back through the bifurcation event, making a checkpoint irreversible. In particular the S and M checkpoints are regulated by means of special bifurcations called a Hopf bifurcation and an infinite period bifurcation.

Protein Structure Prediction

Protein structure prediction is the prediction of the three-dimensional structure of a protein from its amino acid sequence — that is, the prediction of its secondary, tertiary, and quaternary structure from its primary structure. Structure prediction is fundamentally different from the inverse problem of protein design. Protein structure prediction is one of the most important goals pursued by bioinformatics and theoretical chemistry; it is highly important in medicine (for example, in drug design) and biotechnology (for example, in the design of novel enzymes). Every two years, the performance of current methods is assessed in the CASP experiment (Critical Assessment of Techniques for Protein Structure Prediction).

Secondary Structure

Secondary structure prediction is a set of techniques in bioinformatics that aim to predict the local secondary structures of proteins and RNA sequences based only on knowledge of their primary structure - amino acid or nucleotide sequence, respectively. For proteins, a prediction consists of assigning regions of the amino acid sequence as likely alpha helices, beta strands (often noted as "extended" conformations), or turns. The success of a prediction is determined by comparing it to the results of the DSSP algorithm applied to the crystal structure of the protein; for nucleic acids, it may be determined from the hydrogen bonding pattern. Specialized algorithms have been developed for the detection of specific well-defined patterns such as transmembrane helices and coiled coils in proteins, or canonical microRNA structures in RNA.

The best modern methods of secondary structure prediction in proteins reach about 80% accuracy; this high accuracy allows the use of the predictions in fold recognition and ab initio protein structure prediction, classification of structural motifs, and refinement of sequence alignments. The accuracy of current protein secondary structure prediction methods is assessed in weekly benchmarks such as LiveBench and EVA.

Background

Early methods of secondary structure prediction, introduced in the 1960s and early 1970s, focused on identifying likely alpha helices and were based mainly on helix-coil transition models. Significantly more accurate predictions that included beta sheets were introduced in the 1970s and relied on statistical assessments based on probability parameters derived from known solved structures. These methods, applied to a single sequence, are typically at most about 60-65% accurate, and often underpredict beta sheets. The evolutionary conservation of secondary structures can be exploited by simultaneously assessing many homologous sequences in a multiple sequence alignment, by calculating the net secondary structure propensity of an aligned column of amino acids. In concert with larger databases of known protein structures and modern machine learning methods such as neural nets and support vector machines, these methods can achieve up 80% overall accuracy in globular proteins. The theoretical upper limit of accuracy is around 90%, partly due to idiosyncrasies in DSSP assignment near the ends of secondary structures, where local conformations vary under native conditions but may be forced to assume a single conformation in crystals due to packing constraints. Limitations are also imposed by secondary structure prediction's inability to account for tertiary structure; for example, a sequence predicted as a likely helix may still be able to adopt a beta-strand conformation if it is located within a beta-sheet region of the protein and its side chains pack well with their neighbours. Dramatic conformational changes related to the protein's function or environment can also alter local secondary structure.

Chou-Fasman Method

The Chou-Fasman method was among the first secondary structure prediction algorithms developed and relies predominantly on probability parameters determined from relative frequencies of each amino acid's appearance in each type of secondary structure. The original Chou-Fasman parameters, determined from the small sample of structures solved in the mid-1970s, produce poor results compared to modern methods, though the parameterization has been updated since it was first published. The Chou-Fasman method is roughly 50-60% accurate in predicting secondary structures.

GOR Method

The GOR method, named for the three scientists who developed it - *G*arnier, *O*sguthorpe, and *R*obson - is an information theory-based method developed not long after Chou-Fasman. It uses a more powerful probabilistic techniques of Bayesian inference. The method is a specific optimized application of mathematics and algorithms developed in a series of papers by Robson and colleagues, eg. and). The GOR method is capable of continued extension by such principles, and has gone through several versions. The GOR method takes into account not only the probability of each amino acid having a particular secondary structure, but also the conditional probability of the amino acid assuming each structure given the contributions of its neighbours (it does not assume that the neighbours have that same structure). The approach is both more sensitive and more accurate than that of Chou and Fasman because amino acid structural propensities are only strong for a small number of amino acids such as proline and glycine. Weak contributions from each of many neighbours can add up to strong effect overall. The original GOR method was roughly 65% accurate and is dramatically more successful in predicting alpha helices than beta sheets, which it frequently mispredicted as loops or disorganized regions.. Later GOR methods considered also pairs of amino acids, significantly improving performance. The major difference from the following technique is perhaps that the weights in an implied network of contributing terms are assigned *a priori*, from statistical analysis of proteins of known structure, not by feedback to optimize agreement with a training set of such.

Machine Learning

Neural network methods use training sets of solved structures to identify common sequence motifs associated with particular arrangements of secondary structures. These methods are over 70% accurate in their predictions, although beta strands are still often underpredicted due to the lack of three-dimensional structural information that would allow assessment of hydrogen bonding patterns that can promote formation of the extended conformation required for the presence of a complete beta sheet.

Support vector machines have proven particularly useful for predicting the locations of turns, which are difficult to identify with statistical methods. The requirement of relatively small training sets has also been cited as an advantage to avoid overfitting to existing structural data.

Extensions of machine learning techniques attempt to predict more fine-grained local properties of proteins, such as backbone dihedral angles in unassigned regions. Both SVMs and neural networks have been applied to this problem.

Other Improvements

It is reported that in addition to the protein sequence, secondary structure formation depends on other factors. For example, it is reported that secondary structure tendencies depend also on local environment , solvent accessibility of residues , protein structural class , and even the organism from which the proteins are obtained. Based on such observations, some studies have shown that secondary structure prediction can be improved by addition of information about protein structural class, solvent accessibility and also contact number of residues.

Sequence covariation methods rely on the existence of a data set composed of multiple homologous RNA sequences with related but dissimilar sequences. These methods analyse the covariation of individual base sites in evolution; maintenance at two widely separated sites of a pair of base-pairing nucleotides indicates the presence of a structurally required hydrogen bond between those positions. The general problem of pseudoknot prediction has been shown to be NP-complete.

Tertiary Structure

The practical role of protein structure prediction is now more important than ever. Massive amounts of protein sequence data are produced by modern large-scale DNA sequencing efforts such as the Human Genome Project. Despite community-wide efforts in structural genomics, the output of experimentally determined protein structures—typically by time-consuming and relatively expensive X-ray crystallography or NMR spectroscopy—is lagging far behind the output of protein sequences. The protein structure prediction remains an extremely difficult and unresolved undertaking. The two main problems are calculation of protein free energy and finding the global minimum of this energy. A protein structure prediction method must explore the space of possible protein structures which is astronomically large. These problems can be partially bypassed in "comparative" or homology modelling and fold recognition methods, when the search space is pruned by the assumption that the protein in question adopts a structure that is close to the experimentally determined structure of another homologous protein. On the other hand, the *de novo* or ab initio protein structure prediction methods must explicitly resolve these problems.

Ab Initio Protein Modelling

Ab initio- or *de novo-* protein modelling methods seek to build three-dimensional protein models "from scratch", i.e., based on physical principles rather than (directly) on previously solved structures. There are many possible procedures that either attempt to mimic protein folding or apply some stochastic method to search possible solutions (i.e., global optimization of a suitable energy function). These procedures tend to require vast computational resources, and have thus only been carried out for tiny proteins. To predict protein structure *de novo* for larger proteins will require better algorithms and larger computational resources like those afforded by either powerful supercomputers (such as Blue Gene or MDGRAPE-3) or distributed computing (such as Folding@home, the Human Proteome Folding Project and Rosetta@Home). Although these computational barriers are vast, the potential benefits of structural genomics (by predicted or experimental methods) make *ab initio* structure prediction an active research field.

As an intermediate step towards predicted protein structures, contact map predictions have been proposed.

Comparative Protein Modelling

Comparative protein modelling uses previously solved structures as starting points, or templates. This is effective because it appears that although the number of actual proteins is vast, there is a limited set of tertiary structural motifs to which most proteins belong. It has been suggested that there are only around 2,000 distinct protein folds in nature, though there are many millions of different proteins.

These methods may also be split into two groups :

Homology modelling : is based on the reasonable assumption that two homologous proteins will share very similar structures. Because a protein's fold is more evolutionarily conserved than its amino acid sequence, a target sequence can be modelled with reasonable accuracy on a very distantly related template, provided that the relationship between target and template can be discerned through sequence alignment. It has been suggested that the primary bottleneck in comparative modelling arises from difficulties in alignment rather than from errors in structure prediction given a known-good alignment. Unsurprisingly, homology modelling is most accurate when the target and template have similar sequences.

Protein threading : scans the amino acid sequence of an unknown structure against a database of solved structures. In each case, a scoring function is used to assess the compatibility of the sequence to the structure, thus yielding possible three-dimensional models. This type of method is also known as 3D-1D fold recognition due to its compatibility analysis between three-dimensional structures and linear protein sequences. This method has also given rise to methods performing an inverse folding search by evaluating the compatibility of a given structure with a large database of sequences, thus predicting which sequences have the potential to produce a given fold.

Side Chain Geometry Prediction

Accurate packing of the amino acid side chains represents a separate problem. Methods that specifically address the problem of predicting side chain geometry include dead-end elimination and the self-consistent mean field methods. The side chain conformations with low energy are usually determined on the rigid polypeptide backbone and using a set of discrete side chain conformations known as "rotamers" or a "conformational isomerism". The methods attempt to identify the set of rotamers that minimize the model's overall energy.

These methods use rotamer libraries, the collections of rotamers (favourable multi-angle conformations) for each residue type in proteins. Rotamer libraries may contain information about the conformation, its frequency, and the variance about mean dihedral angles, which can be used in sampling. Rotamer libraries are derived from structural bioinformatics or other statistical analysis of side-chain conformations in known experimental structures of proteins, such as by clustering the observed conformations for tetrahedral carbons near the staggered (60°, 180°, -60°) values. Rotamer libraries can be backbone-independent, secondary-structure-dependent, or backbone-dependent. Backbone-independent rotamer libraries make no reference to backbone conformation, and are calculated from all available side chains of a certain type (for instance, the first example of a rotamer library, done by Ponder and Richards at Yale in 1987). Secondary-structure-dependent libraries present different dihedral angles and/or rotamer frequencies for a-helix, b-sheet, or coil secondary structures. Backbone-dependent rotamer libraries present conformations and/or frequencies dependent on the local backbone conformation as defined by the backbone dihedral angles f and y, regardless of secondary structure. The modern versions of these "libraries" as used in most software are presented as multidimensional distributions of probability or frequency, where the peaks correspond to the dihedral-angle conformations considered as individual rotamers in the lists. Some versions are especially sensitive to the prohibited regions in that conformational space and are used primarily for structure validation , while others emphasize relative frequencies in the favourable regions and are the form used primarily for structure prediction, such as the Dunbrack rotamer "libraries".

The side chain packing methods are most useful for analyzing the protein's hydrophobic core, where side chains are more closely packed; they have more difficulty addressing the looser constraints and higher flexibility of surface residues, which often occupy multiple rotamer conformations rather than just one.

Prediction of Structural Classes

Statistical methods have been developed for predicting structural classes of proteins based on their amino acid composition, pseudo amino acid composition and functional domain composition.

Quaternary Structure

In the case of complexes of two or more proteins, where the structures of the proteins are known or can be predicted with high accuracy, protein–protein docking methods can be used to predict the structure of the complex. Information of the effect of mutations at specific sites on the affinity of the complex helps to understand the complex structure and to guide docking methods.

Software

Modeller is a popular software tool for producing homology models using methodology derived from NMR spectroscopy data processing. SwissModel provides an automated web server for basic homology modelling.

I-tasser is the best server for protein structure prediction according to the 2006 2008 CASP experiments (CASP7 and CASP8).

HHpred, bioinfo.pl, Robetta, and Phyre are widely used servers for protein structure prediction. HHsearch is a free software package for protein threading and remote homology detection.

RAPTOR (software) is a protein threading software that is based on integer programming. The basic algorithm for threading is described in and is fairly straightforward to implement. Abalone is a Molecular Dynamics program for folding simulations with explicit or implicit water models.

TIP is a knowledgebase of STRUCTFAST models and precomputed similarity relationships between sequences, structures, and binding sites. Several distributed computing projects concerning protein structure prediction have also been implemented, such as the Folding@home, Rosetta@home, Human Proteome Folding Project, Predictor@home, and TANPAKU.

The Foldit program seeks to investigate the pattern-recognition and puzzle-solving abilities inherent to the human mind in order to create more successful computer protein structure prediction software. Computational approaches provide a fast alternative route to antibody structure prediction. Recently developed antibody F_V region high resolution structure prediction algorithms, like RosettaAntibody, have been shown to generate high resolution homology models which have been used for successful docking. Reviews of software for structure prediction can be found at. The progress and challenges in protein structure prediction has been reviewed in Zhang 2008.

Automatic Structure Prediction Servers

CASP, which stands for Critical Assessment of Techniques for Protein Structure Prediction, is a community-wide experiment for protein structure prediction taking place every two years since 1994. CASP provides users and research groups with an opportunity to assess the quality of available methods and automatic servers for protein structure prediction. Official results for automatic structure prediction servers in the CASP7 benchmark (2006) are discussed by Battey *et al.*. Official CASP8 results are available for automatic servers and for human and server predictors. Unofficial results for automatic servers of the 2008 CASP8 benchmark are summarized on several lab websites and ranked according to slightly varying criteria: Zhang lab, Grishin lab, McGuffin lab, Baker lab, and Cheng lab.

Human Biological Systems

Brain Model

The Blue Brain Project is an attempt to create a synthetic brain by reverse-engineering the mammalian brain down to the molecular level. The aim of the project, founded in May 2005 by the Brain and Mind Institute of the *Ecole Polytechnique* in Lausanne, Switzerland, is to study the brain's architectural and functional principles. The project is headed by the Institute's director, Henry Markram. Using a Blue Gene supercomputer running Michael Hines's NEURON software, the simulation does not consist simply of an artificial neural network, but involves a partially biologically realistic model of neurons. It is hoped by its proponents that it will eventually shed light on the nature of consciousness. There are a number of sub-projects, including the Cajal Blue Brain, coordinated by the Supercomputing and Visualization Centre of Madrid (CeSViMa), and others run by universities and independent laboratories in the UK, U.S., and Israel.

Model of the Immune System

The last decade has seen the emergence of a growing number of simulations of the immune system.

Simulated Growth of Plants

The simulated growth of plants is a significant task in of systems biology and mathematical biology, which seeks to reproduce plant morphology with computer software. Electronic trees (e-trees) usually use L-systems to simulate growth. L-systems are very important in the field of complexity science and A-life. A universally accepted system for describing changes in plant morphology at the cellular or modular level has yet to be devised. The most widely implemented tree-generating algorithms are described in the papers "Creation and Rendering of Realistic Trees", and Real-Time Tree Rendering.

The realistic modelling of plant growth is of high value to biology, but also for computer games.

Theory + Algorithms

A biologist, Aristid Lindenmayer (1925–1989) worked with yeast and filamentous fungi and studied the growth patterns of various types of algae, such as the blue/green bacteria *Anabaena catenula*. Originally the L-systems were devised to provide a formal description of the development of such simple multicellular organisms, and to illustrate the neighbourhood relationships between plant cells. Later on, this system was extended to describe higher plants and complex branching structures. Central to L-systems, is the notion of rewriting, where the basic idea is to define complex objects by successively replacing parts of a simple object using a set of rewriting rules or productions.

The rewriting can be carried out recursively. L-Systems are also closely related to Koch curves.

Environmental Interaction

A challenge for plant simulations is to consistently integrate environmental factors, such as surrounding plants, obstructions, water and mineral availability, and lighting conditions is to build virtual/ environments with as many parameters as computationally feasible, thereby, not only simulating the growth of the plant, but also the environment it is growing within, and, in fact, whole ecosystems. Changes in resource availability influence plant growth, which in turn results in a change of resource availability. Powerful models and powerful hardware will be necessary to effectively simulate these recursive interactions of recursive structures.

Ecosystem Model

Ecosystem models, or ecological models, are mathematical representations of ecosystems. Typically they simplify complex foodwebs down to their major components or trophic levels, and quantify these as either numbers of organisms, biomass or the inventory/ concentration of some pertinent chemical element (for instance, carbon or a nutrient species such as nitrogen or phosphorus).

Overview

Complexity

Ecosystem models are a development of theoretical ecology that aim to characterise the major dynamics of ecosystems, both to synthesise the understanding of such systems and to allow predictions of their behaviour (in general terms, or in response to particular changes).

Because of the complexity of ecosystems (in terms of numbers of species/ecological interactions), ecosystem models typically simplify the systems they are studying to a limited number of pragmatic components. These may be particular species of interest, or may be broad functional types such as autotrophs, heterotrophs or saprotrophs. In biogeochemistry, ecosystem models usually include representations of non-living "resources" such as nutrients, which are consumed by (and may be depleted by) living components of the model.

This simplification is driven by a number of factors:

- Ignorance: while understood in broad outline, the details of a particular foodweb may not be known; this applies both to identifying relevant species, and to the functional responses linking them (which are often extremely difficult to quantify)

- Computation: practical constraints on simulating large numbers of ecological elements; this is particularly true when ecosystem models are embedded within other spatially-resolved models (such as physical models of terrain or ocean bodies, or idealised models such as cellular automata or coupled map lattices)
- Understanding: depending upon the nature of the study, complexity can confound the analysis of an ecosystem model; the more interacting components a model has, the less straightforward it is to extract and separate causes and consequences; this is compounded when uncertainty about components obscures the accuracy of a simulation.

Structure

The process of simplification described above typically reduces an ecosystem to a small number of state variables. Depending upon the system under study, these may represent ecological components in terms of numbers of discrete individuals or quantify the component more continuously as a measure of the total biomass of all organisms of that type, often using a common model currency (e.g. mass of carbon per unit area/volume).

The components are then linked together by mathematical functions that describe the nature of the relationships between them. For instance, in models which include predator-prey relationships, the two components are usually linked by some function that relates total prey captured to the populations of both predators and prey. Deriving these relationships is often extremely difficult given habitat heterogeneity, the details of component behavioral ecology (including issues such as perception, foraging behaviour), and the difficulties involved in unobtrusively studying these relationships under field conditions.

Typically relationships are derived statistically or heuristically. For example, some standard functional forms describing these relationships are linear, quadratic, hyperbolic or sigmoid functions. The latter two are known in ecology as type II and type III responses, named by C. S. Holling in early, groundbreaking work on predation in mammals. Both describe relationships in which a linkage between components saturates at some maximum rate (e.g. above a certain concentration of prey organisms, predators cannot catch any more per unit time). Some ecological interactions are derived explicitly from the biochemical processes that underlie them; for instance, nutrient processing by an organism may saturate because of either a limited number of binding sites on the organism's exterior surface or the rate of diffusion of nutrient across the boundary layer surrounding the organism.

After establishing the components to be modelled and the relationships between them, another important factor in ecosystem model structure is the representation of space used. Historically, models have often ignored the confounding issue of space, utilising zero-dimensional approaches, such as ordinary differential equations. With increases in computational power, models which incorporate space are increasingly used (e.g. partial differential equations, cellular automata). This inclusion of space permits dynamics not present in non-spatial frameworks, and illuminates processes that lead to pattern formation in ecological systems.

Examples

One of the earliest, and most well-known, ecological models is the predator-prey model of Alfred J. Lotka (1925) and Vito Volterra (1926). This model takes the form of a pair of ordinary differential equations, one representing a prey species, the other its predator.

$$\frac{dX}{dt} = \alpha.X - \beta.X.Y$$

$$\frac{dY}{dt} = \gamma.\beta.XY - \gamma.Y$$

Volterra originally devised the model to explain fluctuations in fish and shark populations observed in the Adriatic Sea after the First World War (when fishing was curtailed). However, the equations have subsequently been applied more generally. Although simple, they illustrate some of the salient features of ecological models: modelled biological populations experience growth, interact with other populations (as either predators, prey or competitors) and suffer mortality.

Mathematical Modelling of Infectious Disease

It is possible to mathematically model the progress of most infectious diseases to discover the likely outcome of an epidemic or to help manage them by vaccination. This article uses some basic assumptions and some simple mathematics to find parameters for various infectious diseases and to use those parameters to make useful calculations about the effects of a mass vaccination programme.

History

Early pioneers in infectious disease modelling were William Hamer and Ronald Ross, who in the early twentieth century applied the law of mass action to explain epidemic behaviour.

Lowell Reed and Wade Hampton Frost developed the Reed-Frost epidemic model which described the relationship between susceptible, infected and immune individuals in a population.

Concepts

R_0, the basic reproduction number :

The average number of other individuals each infected individual will infect in a population that has no immunity to the disease.

S : The proportion of the population who are susceptible to the disease (neither immune nor infected).

A :The average age at which the disease is contracted in a given population.

L: The average life expectancy in a given population.

Assumptions

- We assume a rectangular age distribution, such as that which is typically found in developed countries where there is a low infant mortality and much of the population lives to the life expectancy. In developed countries this assumption is often well justified.
- We also assume homogeneous mixing of the population, i.e., individuals of the population under scrutiny assort and make contact at random and do not mix mostly in a smaller subgroup. This assumption is rarely justified, when dealing with a country such as the UK, because most people in London, say, only make contact with other Londoners. If we deal only with London, then there will be smaller subgroups such as the Turkish community or teenagers (just to give two examples) who will mix with each other more than people outside their group. However, homogeneous mixing is a standard assumption to make the mathematics tractable.

Whenever we are modelling anything mathematically, whether in epidemiology or otherwise, we would be wise to remember that a mathematical model is only as good as the assumptions on which it is based. If a model makes predictions which are out of line with observed results and the mathematics is correct, we must go back and change our initial assumptions in order to make the model useful.

The Endemic Steady State

An infectious disease is said to be endemic when it can be sustained in a population without the need for external inputs.

This means that, on average, each infected person is infecting *exactly* one other person (any more and the number of people infected will grow exponentially and there will be an epidemic, any less and the disease will die out). In mathematical terms, that is:

$$R_0 \times S = 1.$$

The basic reproduction number (R_0) of the disease, assuming everyone is susceptible, multiplied by the proportion of the population that is actually susceptible (S) must be one (since those who are not susceptible do not feature in our calculations as they cannot contract the disease).

Notice that this relation means that for a disease to be in the endemic steady state, the higher the basic reproduction number, the lower the proportion of the population susceptible must be, and vice versa; a mathematical basis for a result that might have been intuitively obvious.

The first assumption lets us say that everyone in the population lives to age L and then dies. If the average age of infection is A, then on average individuals younger than A are susceptible and those older than A are immune (or infectious). Thus the proportion of the population that is susceptible is given by:

$$S = \frac{A}{L}.$$

But the mathematical definition of the endemic steady state can be rearranged to give:

$$S = \frac{1}{R_0}.$$

And therefore, since things equal to the same thing are equal to each other:

$$\frac{1}{R_0} = \frac{A}{L}$$

$$R_0 = \frac{L}{A}.$$

This provides us with a simple way to estimate the parameter R_0 using easily available data.

In a Population with an Exponential Age Distribution

For a population with an exponential age distribution, it turns out that

$$R_0 = 1 + \frac{L}{A}.$$

The mathematics required to calculate this is a little more complicated than that above, and thus beyond the scope of this article. However, this does allow you to work out the basic reproduction number of a disease given A and L in either type of population distribution.

Infectious Disease Dynamics

In recent years it has become obvious that there is a need to accommodate the growing integration of quantitative methods with the increasing volume of data being generated on host-pathogen interactions. This has resulted in a growing body of research covering quantitative or theoretical studies of the population dynamics, structure and evolution of infectious diseases of plants and animals, including humans.

Specific topics in this area include:

- transmission, spread and control of infection
- epidemiological networks
- spatial epidemiology
- persistence of pathogens within hosts
- intra-host dynamics
- immuno-epidemiology
- virulence
- Strain (biology) structure and interactions
- antigenic shift
- phylodynamics
- pathogen population genetics
- evolution and spread of resistance
- role of host genetic factors
- statistical and mathematical tools and innovations
- role and identification of infection reservoirs.

The Mathematics of Mass Vaccination

If the proportion of the population that is immune exceeds the herd immunity level for the disease, then the disease can no longer persist in the population. Thus, if this level can be exceeded by vaccination, the disease can be eliminated. An example of this being successfully achieved worldwide is the global eradication of smallpox, with the last wild case in 1977. Currently, the WHO is carrying out a similar campaign of vaccination in an attempt to eradicate polio.

The herd immunity level will be denoted q. Recall that, for a stable state:

$$R_0.S = 1$$

S will be $(1 - q)$, since q is the proportion of the population that is immune and $q + S$ must equal one (since in this simplified model, everyone is either susceptible or immune). Then:

$$R_0.(1-q) = 1;$$

$$1-q = \frac{1}{R_0},$$

$$q = 1 - \frac{1}{R_0}.$$

Remember that this is the threshold level. If the proportion of immune individuals *exceeds* this level due to a mass vaccination programme, the disease will die out.

We have just calculated the critical immunisation threshold (denoted q_c). It is the minimum proportion of the population that must be immunised at birth (or close to birth) in order for the infection to die out in the population.

$$qc = 1 - \frac{1}{R_0}$$

When a mass vaccination programme cannot exceed the herd immunity

If the vaccine used is insufficiently effective or the required coverage cannot be reached (for example due to popular resistance) the programme may not be able to exceed q_c. Such a programme can, however, disturb the balance of the infection without eliminating it, often causing unforeseen problems.

Suppose that a proportion of the population q (where $q < q_c$) is immunised at birth against an infection with $R_0>1$. The vaccination programme changes R_0 to R_q where

$$R_q = R_0(1-q)$$

This change occurs simply because there are now fewer susceptibles in the population who can be infected. R_q is simply R_0 minus those that would normally be infected but that cannot be now since they are immune. As a consequence of this lower basic reproduction number, the average age of infection A will also change to some new value A_q in those who have been left unvaccinated.

Recall the relation that linked R_0, A and L. Assuming that life expectancy has not changed, now:

$$R_q = \frac{L}{A_q},$$

$$A_q = \frac{L}{R_q},$$

$$A_q = \frac{L}{R_0(1-q)}.$$

But $R_0 = L/A$ so:

$$A_q = \frac{L}{(L/A)(1-q)},$$

$$A_q = \frac{AL}{L(1-q)},$$

$$A_q = \frac{A}{1-q}.$$

Thus the vaccination programme will produce an increase in the average age of infection, another mathematical justification for a result that might have been intuitively obvious. Unvaccinated individuals now experience a reduced force of infection due to the presence of the vaccinated group.

However, it is important to consider this effect when vaccinating against diseases which increase in severity with age. A vaccination programme against such a disease that does not exceed q_c may cause more deaths and complications than there were before the programme was brought into force as individuals will be catching the disease later in life. These unforeseen outcomes of a vaccination programme are called perverse effects.

When a Mass Vaccination Programme Exceeds the Herd Immunity

If a vaccination programme causes the proportion of immune individuals in a population to exceed the critical threshold for a significant length of time, transmission of the infectious disease in that population will gradually come to a halt. This is known as elimination of the infection and is different from eradication.

Elimination

Interruption of endemic transmission of an infectious disease, which occurs if each infected individual infects less than one other and is achieved by maintaining vaccination coverage to keep the proportion of immune individuals above the critical immunisation threshold.

Eradication

Reduction of infective organisms in the wild worldwide to zero. So far, this has only been achieved for smallpox. To get to eradication, elimination in all world regions must first be progressed through.

Epidemic Model

An Epidemic model is a simplified means of describing the transmission of communicable disease through individuals.

Introduction

The outbreak and spread of disease has been questioned and studied for many years. The ability to make predictions about diseases could enable scientists to evaluate inoculation or isolation plans and may have a significant effect on the mortality rate of a particular epidemic. The modelling of infectious diseases is a tool which has been used to study the mechanisms by which diseases spread, to predict the future course of an outbreak and to evaluate strategies to control an epidemic (Daley & Gani, 2005).

The first scientist who systematically tried to quantify causes of death was John Graunt in his book *Natural and Political Observations made upon the Bills of Mortality*, in 1662. The bills he studied were listings of numbers and causes of deaths published weekly. Graunt's analysis of causes of death is considered the beginning of the "theory of competing risks" which according to Daley and Gani is "a theory that is now well established among modern epidemiologists".

The earliest account of mathematical modelling of spread of disease was carried out in 1766 by Daniel Bernoulli. Trained as a physician, Bernoulli created a mathematical model to defend the practice of inoculating against smallpox (Hethcote, 2000). The calculations from this model showed that universal inoculation against smallpox would increase the life expectancy from 26 years 7 months to 29 years 9 months. Following Bernoulli, other physicians contributed to modern mathematical epidemiology. Among the most acclaimed of these were A. G. McKendrick and W. O. Kermack, whose paper *A Contribution to the Mathematical Theory of Epidemics* was published in 1927. A simple deterministic (compartmental) model was formulated in this paper. The model was successful in predicting the Behaviour of outbreaks very similar to that observed in many recorded epidemics (Brauer & Castillo-Chavez, 2001).

Types of Epidemic Models

Stochastic

"Stochastic" means being or having a random variable. A stochastic model is a tool for estimating probability distributions of potential outcomes by allowing for random variation in one or more inputs over time. Stochastic models depend on the chance variations in risk of exposure, disease and other illness dynamics. They are used when these fluctuations are important, as in small populations.

Deterministic

When dealing with large populations, as in the case of tuberculosis, deterministic or compartmental mathematical models are used. In the deterministic model, individuals in the population are assigned to different subgroups or compartments, each representing a specific stage of the epidemic. Letters such as M, S, E, I, and R are often used to represent different stage.

The transition rates from one class to another are mathematically expressed as derivatives, hence the model is formulated using differential equations. While building such models, it must be assumed that the population size in a compartment is differentiable with respect to time and that the epidemic process is deterministic. In other words, the changes in population of a compartment can be calculated using only the history used to develop the model.

Another approach is through discrete analysis on a lattice (such as a two-dimensional square grid), where the updating is done through asynchronous single-site updates (Kinetic Monte Carlo) or synchronous updating (Cellular Automata). The lattice approach enables inhomogeneities and clustering to be taken into account. Lattice systems are usually studied through computer simulation, and are discussed in the Wikipedia page Epidemic models on lattices.

Terminology

The following is a summary of the notation used in this and the next sections.

- M — Passively Immune Infants
- S — Susceptibles
- E — Exposed Individuals in the Latent Period
- I — Infectives
- R — Removed with Immunity
- b — Contact Rate
- m — Average Death Rate
- B — Averate Birth Rate
- 1/e — Average Latent Period
- 1/g — Average Infectious Period
- R_0 — Basic Reproduction Number
- N — Total Population
- *f* — Average Loss of Immunity Rate of Recovered Individuals
- d — Average Temporary Immunity Period.

Deterministic Compartmental Models

The SIR Model

In 1927, W. O. Kermack and A. G. McKendrick created a model in which they considered a fixed population with only three compartments, susceptible: S(t), infected, I(t), and recovered, R(t).The compartments used for this model consist of three classes:

- S(t) is used to represent the number of individuals not yet infected with the disease at time t, or those susceptible to the disease
- I(t) denotes the number of individuals who have been infected with the disease and are capable of spreading the disease to those in the susceptible category

- R(t) is the compartment used for those individuals who have been infected and then recovered from the disease. Those in this category are not able to be infected again or to transmit the infection to others.

The flow of this model may be considered as follows:

$$S \rightarrow L \rightarrow S$$

Using a fixed population, N = S(t) + I(t) + R(t), Kermack and McKendrick derived the following equations:

$$\frac{dS}{dT} = -\beta SI$$

$$\frac{dI}{dT} = \beta SI - \gamma I$$

$$\frac{dR}{dT} = \gamma I$$

Several assumptions were made in the formulation of these equations:

First, an individual in the population must be considered as having an equal probability as every other individual of contracting the disease with a rate of b, which is considered the contact or infection rate of the disease. Therefore, an infected individual makes contact and is able to transmit the disease with bN others per unit time and the fraction of contacts by an infected with a susceptible is S/N. The number of new infections in unit time per infective then is (bN)(S/N), giving the rate of new infections (or those leaving the susceptible category) as (bN)(S/N)I = bSI. For the second and third equations, consider the population leaving the susceptible class as equal to the number entering the infected class. However, a number equal to the fraction (g which represents the mean recovery rate, or 1/g the mean infective period) of infectives are leaving this class per unit time to enter the removed class. These processes which occur simultaneously are referred to as the Law of Mass Action, a widely accepted idea that the rate of contact between two groups in a population is proportional to the size of each of the groups concerned. Finally, it is assumed that the rate of infection and recover is much faster than the time scale of births and deaths and therefore, these factors are ignored in this model.

The SIR Model with Births and Deaths

Using the case of measles, for example, there is an arrival of new susceptible individuals into the population. For this type of situation births and deaths must be included in the model. The following differential equations represent this model:

$$\frac{dS}{dT} = -\beta SI + \mu(N - S)$$

$$\frac{dI}{dT} = \beta SI - \gamma I - \mu I$$

$$\frac{dR}{dT} = \gamma I - \mu R$$

The SIS Model with Births and Deaths

The SIS model can be easily derived from the SIR model by simply considering that the individuals recover with no immunity to the disease, that is, individuals are immediately susceptible once they have recovered.

$$S \rightarrow L \rightarrow S$$

Removing the equation representing the recovered population from the SIR model and adding those removed from the infected population into the susceptible population gives the following differential equations:

$$\frac{dS}{dT} = -\beta SI + \mu(N - S) + \gamma I$$

$$\frac{dI}{dT} = \beta SI - \gamma I - \mu I$$

The SIRS Model

This model is simply an extension of the SIR model as we will see from its construction.

$$S \rightarrow L \rightarrow R \rightarrow S$$

The only difference is that it allows members of the recovered class to be free of infection and rejoin the susceptible class.

$$\frac{dS}{dT} = -\beta SI + \mu(N - S) + fR$$

$$\frac{dI}{dT} = \beta SI - \gamma I - \mu I$$

$$\frac{dR}{dT} = \gamma I - \mu R - fR$$

Models with More Compartments

The SEIS Model

The SEIS model takes into consideration the exposed or latent period of the disease, giving an additional compartment, E(t).

$$S \to \varepsilon \to L \to S$$

In this model an infection does not leave a long lasting immunity thus individuals that have recovered return to being susceptible again, moving back into the S(t) compartment. The following differential equations describe this model:

$$\frac{dS}{dT} = B - \beta SI - \mu S + \gamma I$$

$$\frac{dE}{dT} = \beta SI - (\varepsilon - \mu)E$$

$$\frac{dI}{dT} = \varepsilon E - (\gamma + \mu)I$$

The SEIR Model

The SIR model discussed above takes into account only those diseases which cause an individual to be able to infect others immediately upon their infection. Many diseases have what is termed a latent or exposed phase, during which the individual is said to be infected but not infectious.

$$S \to \varepsilon \to L \to R$$

In this model the host population (N) is broken into four compartments: susceptible, exposed, infectious, and recovered, with the numbers of individuals in a compartment, or their densities denoted respectively by S(t), E(t), I(t), R(t), that is N = S(t) + E(t) + I(t) + R(t)

$$\frac{dS}{dT} = B - \beta SI - \mu S$$

$$\frac{dE}{dT} = \beta SI - (\varepsilon + \mu)E$$

$$\frac{dI}{dT} = \varepsilon E - (\gamma + \mu)I$$

$$\frac{dR}{dT} = \gamma I - \mu R$$

The MSIR Model

There are several diseases where an individual is born with a passive immunity from its mother.

$$M \rightarrow S \rightarrow L \rightarrow R$$

To indicate this mathematically, an additional compartment is added, M(t), which results in the following differential equations:

$$\frac{dM}{dT} = B - oMS - \mu S$$

$$\frac{dS}{dT} = oMS - \beta SI - \mu S$$

$$\frac{dI}{dT} = \beta SI - \gamma I - \mu I$$

$$\frac{dR}{dT} = \gamma I - \mu R$$

The MSEIR Model

For the case of a disease, with the factors of passive immunity, and a latency period there is the MSEIR model.

$$M \rightarrow S \rightarrow \varepsilon \rightarrow L \rightarrow R$$

$$\frac{dM}{dT} = B - oMS - \mu M$$

$$\frac{dS}{dT} = oMS - \beta SI - \mu S$$

$$\frac{dE}{dT} = \beta SI - (\varepsilon + \mu)E$$

$$\frac{dI}{dT} = \varepsilon E - (\gamma + \mu)I$$

$$\frac{dR}{dT} = \gamma I - \mu R$$

The MSEIRS Model

An MSEIRS model is similar to the MSEIR, but the immunity in the R class would be temporary, so that individuals would regain their susceptibility when the temporary immunity ended.

$$M \rightarrow S \rightarrow \varepsilon \rightarrow L \rightarrow R \rightarrow S$$

Reproduction Number

Basic Reproduction Number

In epidemiology, the basic reproduction number (sometimes called basic reproductive rate or basic reproductive ratio) of an infection is the mean number of secondary cases a typical single infected case will cause in a population with no immunity to the disease in the absence of interventions to control the infection. It is often denoted R_0. This metric is useful because it helps determine whether or not an infectious disease will spread through a population. The roots of the basic reproduction concept can be traced through the work of Alfred Lotka, Ronald Ross, and others, but its first modern application in epidemiology was by George MacDonald in 1952, who constructed population models of the spread of malaria.

Values of R_0 of well-known infectious diseases

Disease	*Transmission*	R_0
Measles	Airborne	12–18
Pertussis	Airborne droplet	12–17
Diphtheria	Saliva	6–7
Smallpox	Social contact	5–7
Polio	Fecal-oral route	5–7
Rubella	Airborne droplet	5–7
Mumps	Airborne droplet	4–7
HIV/AIDS	Sexual contact	2–5
SARS	Airborne droplet	2–5
Influenza	Airborne droplet	2–3

When:

$R_0 < 1$

the infection will die out in the long run (provided infection rates are constant). But if:

$R_0 > 1$

The infection will be able to spread in a population. Large values of R_0 may indicate the possibility of a major epidemic.

Generally, the larger the value of R_0, the harder it is to control the epidemic. In particular, the proportion of the population that needs to be vaccinated to prevent sustained spread of the infection is given by $1 - 1/R_0$. The basic reproductive rate is affected by several factors including the duration of infectivity of affected patients, the infectiousness of the organism, and the number of susceptible people in the population that the affected patients are in contact with.

Other Uses

R_0 is also used as a measure of individual reproductive success in population ecology, evolutionary invasion analysis and life history theory. It represents the average number of offspring produced over the lifetime of an individual (under ideal conditions).

For simple population models, R_0 can be calculated, provided an explicit decay rate (or "death rate") is given. In this case, the reciprocal of the decay rate (usually $1/d$) gives the average lifetime of an individual. When multiplied by the average number of offspring per individual per timestep (the "birth rate" b), this gives $R_0 = b / d$. For more complicated models that have variable growth rates (e.g. because of self-limitation or dependence on food densities), the maximum growth rate should be used.

Limitations of R_0

When calculated from mathematical models, particularly ordinary differential equations, what is often claimed to be R_0 is, in fact, simply a threshold, not the average number of secondary infections. There are many methods used to derive such a threshold from a mathematical model, but few of them always give the true value of R_0. This is particularly problematic if there are intermediate vectors between hosts, such as malaria.

What these thresholds will do is determine whether a disease will die out (if $R_0 < 1$) or become endemic (if $R_0 > 1$), but they generally can not compare different diseases.

Methods include the survival function, rearranging the largest eigenvalue of the Jacobian matrix, the next-generation method , calculations from the intrinsic growth rate , existence of the endemic equilibrium, the number of susceptibles at the endemic equilibrium, the average age of infection and the final size equation. Few of these methods agree with one another, even when starting with the same system of differential equations. Even fewer actually calculate the average number of secondary infections. Since R_0 is rarely observed in the field and is usually calculated via a mathematical model, this severely limits its usefulness.

Chapter 5

Genetic Genealogy

Genetic genealogy is the application of genetics to traditional genealogy. Genetic genealogy involves the use of genealogical DNA testing to determine the level of genetic relationship between individuals.

History

The investigation of surnames in genetics can be said to go back to George Darwin, a son of Charles Darwin. In 1875, George Darwin used surnames to estimate the frequency of first-cousin marriages and calculated the expected incidence of marriage between people of the same surname (isonymy). He arrived at a figure between 2.25% and 4.5% for cousin-marriage in the population of Great Britain, with the upper classes being on the high end and the general rural population on the low end. (His parents, Charles Darwin and Emma Wedgwood, were first cousins.) This simple study was innovative for its era. The next stimulus toward using genetics to study family history had to wait until the 1990s, when certain locations on the Y chromosome were identified as being useful for tracing male-to-male inheritance.

Dr. Karl Skorecki, a Canadian nephrologist of Ashkenazi parentage, noticed that a Sephardic fellow-congregant who was a Kohen like himself had completely different physical features. According to Jewish tradition, all Kohanim are descended from the priest Aaron, brother of Moses. Skorecki reasoned that if Kohanim were indeed the descendants of only one man, they should have a common set of genetic markers and should perhaps preserve some family resemblance to each other.

To test that hypothesis, he contacted Professor Michael Hammer of the University of Arizona, a researcher in molecular genetics and pioneer in Y chromosome research. Their report in the *Nature* in 1997 sent shock waves through the worlds of science and religion. A particular marker was indeed more likely to be present in Jewish men from the priestly tradition than in the general Jewish population. It was apparently true that a common descent had been strictly preserved for thousands of years. Moreover, the data showed that there were very few "non-paternity events".

The first to test the new methodology in general surname research was Bryan Sykes, a molecular biologist at Oxford University. His study of the Sykes surname obtained valid results by looking at only four markers on the male chromosome. It pointed the way to genetics becoming a valuable assistant in the service of genealogy and history.

In April 2000, Family Tree DNA began offering the first genetic genealogy tests to the public. This offering marked the first time that a personal theory on the Y chromosome could be tested outside of an academic study. Additionally, Sykes' concept of a surname study, which by this time had been adopted by several other academic researchers outside of Oxford, was expanded into online Surname Projects (an early form of social network) and the effort helped spread knowledge gained through testing to interested genealogists worldwide.

In 2001, Sykes went on to write the popular book *The Seven Daughters of Eve*, which described the seven major haplogroups of European ancestors. In the wake of the book's success, and with the growing availability and affordability of genealogical DNA testing, genetic genealogy as a field began growing rapidly. By 2003, the field of DNA testing of surnames was declared officially to have "arrived" in an article by Jobling and Tyler-Smith in *Nature Reviews Genetics*. The number of firms offering tests, and the number of consumers ordering them, had risen dramatically.

Another milestone in the acceptance of genetic genealogy is the Genographic Project. The Genographic Project is a five-year research study launched in 2005 by the National Geographic Society and IBM, in partnership with the University of Arizona and Family Tree DNA. Although its goals are primarily anthropological, not genealogical, the project's sale by April 2010 of more than 350,000 of its public participation testing kits, which test the general public for either twelve STR markers on the Y chromosome or mutations on the HVR1 region of the mtDNA, has helped increase the visibility of genetic genealogy.

More state-of-the-art commercial laboratories now recommend testing at least 25 markers, since the more markers tested, the more discriminating and powerful the results will be. A 12-marker STR test is usually not discriminating enough to provide conclusive results for a common surname. Genetic laboratories such as Genebase and Family Tree DNA give the option of testing 67 Y-DNA Markers.

Annual sales of genetic genealogical tests for all companies, including the laboratories that support them, are estimated to be in the area of $60 million (2006).

Interpretation

Since the year 2000, dozens of relevant academic papers have been published, and thousands of private test results organised by surname study groups have been made available on the internet. The comparison of results may be complicated by the fact that some laboratories use different testing methods. Apparently differing results from two sources may in fact be identical, and vice-versa.

Uses

Paternal and Maternal Lineages Via DNA Testing

The two most common types of genetic genealogy tests are Y-DNA (paternal line) and mtDNA (maternal line) genealogical DNA tests. Note that Y chromosome and Y-DNA are used interchangeably in this article.

These tests involve the comparison of certain sequences of the DNA of pairs of individuals in order to estimate the probability that they share a common ancestor in a genealogical time frame and, through the use of a Bayesian model published by Bruce Walsh, to estimate the number of generations separating the two individuals from their most recent common ancestor or "mrca".

Y-DNA testing involves short tandem repeat (STR) and, sometimes, single nucleotide polymorphism (SNP) testing of the Y-chromosome. The Y-chromosome is present only in males and reveals information on the strict paternal line. These tests can provide insight into the recent (via STRs) and ancient (via SNPs) genetic ancestry. A Y-chromosome STR test will reveal a haplotype, which should be similar among all male descendants of a male ancestor. SNP tests are used to assign people to a paternal haplogroup, which defines a much larger genetic population.

mtDNA testing involves sequencing or testing the HVR-1 region, HVR-2 region or both. An mtDNA test may also include the additional SNPs needed to assign people to a maternal haplogroup—or even include the complete mtDNA.

Either Y-DNA or mtDNA test results can be compared to the results of others via private or public DNA databases.

Biogeographical and Ethnic Origins

Additional DNA tests exist for determining biogeographical and ethnic origin, but these tests have less relevance for traditional genealogy.

Genetic genealogy has revealed astonishing links between peoples. For instance, it has shown that the ancient Phoenician people were ancestors of much of the present-day population of the island of Malta. Preliminary results from a study by Pierre Zalloua of the American University of Beirut and Spencer Wells, supported by a grant from National Geographic's Committee for Research and Exploration, were published in the October 2004 issue of *National Geographic*. One of the conclusions is that "more than half of the Y chromosome lineages that we see in today's Maltese population could have come in with the Phoenicians."

Human Migration

Genealogical DNA testing methods are also being used on a longer time scale to trace human migratory patterns. For example, they have been used to determine when the first humans came to North America and what path they followed. For several years, a number of researchers and laboratories from around the world have been sampling indigenous populations from around the globe in an effort to map historical human migration patterns. Recently, several projects have been created that are aimed at bringing this science to the public. One example, mentioned in History above, is the National Geographic Society's Genographic Project, which aims to map historical human migration patterns by collecting and analyzing DNA samples from over 100,000 people across five continents. Another example is the DNA Clans Genetic Ancestry Analysis, which measures a person's precise genetic connections to indigenous ethnic groups from around the world.

Typical Customers and Interest Groups

Male DNA testing customers most often start with a Y chromosome test to determine their father's paternal ancestry. Females generally begin with a mitochondrial test to trace their ancient maternal lineage, which males often have tested for the same purpose.

A common consumer goal in purchasing DNA testing services is to acquire quantified, scientific linkage to a specific ancestral group. A compelling example of this motive is found in the expressed desires of some consumers to be proven to have Viking paternal ancestry. In keeping with this marketplace demand, one British DNA testing service, Oxford Ancestors, offers a Y chromosome test purporting to assess whether given males are of "Viking stock." Those whose DNA falls into the designated haplogroup are issued Viking Descendant certificates by the testing service. The same DNA testing company participated in producing a televised documentary, "The Blood of the Vikings," in conjunction with the BBC, which showed how DNA testing could reveal Viking ancestry.

The RootsWeb Genealogy-DNA Internet discussion group has a membership of 750 subscribers from around the world. Some subscribers have had various DNA tests performed and are seeking advice and guidance in interpreting their results. The list also includes administrators of DNA projects that examine surnames, geographic regions, or ethnic groups. The sophistication of subscribers ranges from expert to novice. In some cases, subscribers have been credited with making useful and novel contributions to knowledge in the field of genetic genealogy.

Paternal and Maternal DNA Lineages

Mitochondria are small organelles that lie in the cytoplasm of eukaryotic cells, such as those of humans. Their primary purpose is to provide energy to the cell. Mitochondria are thought to be the vestigial remains of symbiotic bacteria that were once free living. One indication that mitochondria were once free living is that they contain a relatively small circular segment of DNA, called mitochondrial DNA (mtDNA). The overwhelming majority of a human's DNA is contained in chromosomes in the nucleus of the cell, but mtDNA is an exception. Individuals inherit their cytoplasm and the organelles it contains exclusively from their mothers, as these are derived from the ovum (egg cell) only, not from the sperm.

When a mutation arises in mtDNA molecule, the mutation is therefore passed in a direct female line of descent. These rare mutations are derived from copying mistakes—when the DNA is copied it is possible that a single mistake occurs in the DNA sequence, an outcome which is called a single nucleotide polymorphism (SNP).

Human Y chromosomes are male-specific sex chromosomes; nearly all humans that possess a Y chromosome will be morphologically male. Y chromosomes are therefore passed from father to son; although Y chromosomes are situated in the cell nucleus, they only recombine with the X chromosome at the ends of the Y chromosome; the vast majority of the Y chromosome (95%) does not recombine. When mutations (SNPs, and STR copying mistakes) arise in the Y chromosome, they are passed down directly from father to son in a direct male line of descent. The Y-DNA and mtDNA therefore share a certain feature: they both pass down unchanged except for mutations.

The other chromosomes, autosomes and X chromosomes in women, share their genetic material (called crossing over leading to recombination) during meiosis (a special type of cell division that occurs for the purposes of sexual reproduction). Effectively this means that the genetic material from these chromosomes gets mixed up in every generation, and so any new mutations are passed down randomly from parents to offspring. The special feature that both Y-DNA and mtDNA share, above, preserves a "written" record of their mutations because neither DNA gets mixed up or randomized—mutations remain fixed in place on both types of DNA. Furthermore the historical sequence of these mutations can also be inferred. For example, if a set of ten Y chromosomes (derived from ten different men) contains a mutation, A, but only five of these chromosomes contain a second mutation, B, it must be the case that mutation B occurred after mutation A.

Furthermore all ten men who carry the chromosome with mutation A are the direct male line descendants of the same man who was the first to carry this mutation. The first man to carry mutation B was also a direct male line descendant of this man, but is also the direct male line ancestor of all men carrying mutation B. Series of mutations such as this form molecular lineages. Furthermore each SNP mutation may define a set of specific Y chromosomes called a haplogroup.

All men carrying SNP mutation A form a single haplogroup, and all men carrying mutation B are part of this haplogroup, but mutation B (if a SNP) may also define a more recent haplogroup (which is a subgroup or subclade) of its own which men carrying only mutation A do not belong to. Both mtDNA and Y chromosomes or Y-DNA are grouped into lineages and haplogroups; these are often presented as tree-like diagrams.

Benefits

Genetic genealogy gives genealogists a means to check or supplement their genealogy results with information obtained via DNA testing. A positive test match with another individual may:

- provide locations for further genealogical research
- help determine ancestral homeland
- discover living relatives

- validate existing research
- confirm or deny suspected connections between families
- prove or disprove theories regarding ancestry.

Drawbacks

People who resist testing may cite one of the following concerns:

- Cost
- Quality of testing
- Concerns over privacy issues
- Loss of ethnic identity.

Finally, Y-DNA and mtDNA tests each only trace a single lineage (one's father's father's father's etc. lineage or one's mother's mother's mother's etc. lineage). At 10 generations back, an individual has up to 1024 unique ancestors (fewer if ancestor cousins interbred) and a Y-DNA or mtDNA test is only studying one of those ancestors, as well as their descendants and siblings (same sexed siblings for Y-DNA or all siblings for mtDNA). However, most genealogists maintain contact with many cousins (1st, 2nd, 3rd, etc., with different surnames) whose Y-DNA and mtDNA are different, and thus can be encouraged to be tested to find additional ancestral DNA lineages.

Expected Growth

Genetic genealogy is a rapidly growing field. As the cost of testing continues to drop, the number of people being tested continues to increase. The probability of finding a genetic match among the DNA databases should continue to improve. Laboratories and testing firms are engaging in active research and development that will allow for higher confidence intervals and better results interpretation, including historical interpretive reports and customized research.

Genetic Distance among Relatives

Where the genogram or family tree of individuals is known, it can be used to determine the genetic identity between individuals. It is often described as percentage of genetic identity, referring to the fraction of genome inherited from common ancestors, and not actual genomic identity, which is always approximately 99.9% identical from one human to another. One method of calculating this genetic similarity is to do an inbreeding calculation by the path or tabular method and then multiply by 2, because any progeny would have a 1 in 2 risk of actually inheriting the identical alleles from both parents. For instance, a brother/sister relation gives 25% risk for two alleles to be identical by descent.

History of Molecular Biology

The history of molecular biology begins in the 1930s with the convergence of various, previously distinct biological disciplines: biochemistry, genetics, microbiology, and virology. With the hope of understanding life at its most fundamental level, numerous physicists and chemists also took an interest in what would become molecular biology.

In its modern sense, molecular biology attempts to explain the phenomena of life starting from the macromolecular properties that generate them. Two categories of macromolecules in particular are the focus of the molecular biologist: 1) nucleic acids, among which the most famous is deoxyribonucleic acid (or DNA), the constituent of genes, and 2) proteins, which are the active agents of living organisms. One definition of the scope of molecular biology therefore is to characterize the structure, function and relationships between these two types of macromolecules. This relatively limited definition will suffice to allow us to establish a date for the so-called "molecular revolution", or at least to establish a chronology of its most fundamental developments.

General Overview

In its earliest manifestations, molecular biology—the name was coined by Warren Weaver of the Rockefeller Foundation in 1938—was an ideal of physical and chemical explanations of life, rather than a coherent discipline. Following the advent of the Mendelian-chromosome theory of heredity in the 1910s and the maturation of atomic theory and quantum mechanics in the 1920s, such explanations seemed within reach. Weaver and others encouraged (and funded) research at the intersection of biology, chemistry and physics, while prominent physicists such as Niels Bohr and Erwin Schrodinger turned their attention to biological speculation. However, in the 1930s and 1940s it was by no means clear which—if any—cross-disciplinary research would bear fruit; work in colloid chemistry, biophysics and radiation biology, crystallography, and other emerging fields all seemed promising.

In 1940, George Beadle and Edward Tatum demonstrated the existence of a precise relationship between genes and proteins. In the course of their experiments connecting genetics with biochemistry, they switched from the genetics mainstay *Drosophila* to a more appropriate model organism, the fungus *Neurospora*; the construction and exploitation of new model organisms would become a recurring theme in the development of molecular biology. In 1944, Oswald

Avery, working at the Rockefeller Institute of New York, demonstrated that genes are made up of DNA. In 1952, Alfred Hershey and Martha Chase confirmed that the genetic material of the bacteriophage, the virus which infects bacteria, is made up of DNA. In 1953, James Watson and Francis Crick discovered the double helical structure of the DNA molecule. In 1961, Francois Jacob and Jacques Monod hypothesized the existence of an intermediary between DNA and its protein products, which they called messenger RNA. Between 1961 and 1965, the relationship between the information contained in DNA and the structure of proteins was determined: there is a code, the genetic code, which creates a correspondence between the succession of nucleotides in the DNA sequence and a series of amino acids in proteins. At the beginning of the 1960s, Monod and Jacob also demonstrated how certain specific proteins, called regulative proteins, latch onto DNA at the edges of the genes and control the transcription of these genes into messenger RNA; they direct the "expression" of the genes.

The chief discoveries of molecular biology took place in a period of only about twenty-five years. Another fifteen years were required before new and more sophisticated technologies, united today under the name of genetic engineering, would permit the isolation and characterization of genes, in particular those of highly complex organisms.

The Exploration of the Molecular Dominion

If we evaluate the molecular revolution within the context of biological history, it is easy to note that it is the culmination of a long process which began with the first observations through a microscope. The aim of these early researchers was to understand the functioning of living organisms by describing their organization at the microscopic level. From the end of the 18th century, the characterization of the chemical molecules which make up living beings gained increasingly greater attention, along with the birth of physiological chemistry in the 19th century, developed by the German chemist Justus von Liebig and following the birth of biochemistry at the beginning of the 20th, thanks to another German chemist Eduard Buchner. Between the molecules studied by chemists and the tiny structures visible under the optical microscope, such as the cellular nucleus or the chromosomes, there was an obscure zone, "the world of the ignored dimensions," as it was called by the chemical-physicist Wolfgang Ostwald. This world is populated by colloids, chemical compounds whose structure and properties were not well defined.

The successes of molecular biology derived from the exploration of that unknown world by means of the new technologies developed by chemists and physicists: X-ray diffraction, electron microscopy, ultracentrifugization, and electrophoresis. These studies revealed the structure and function of the macromolecules.

A milestone in that process was the work of Dr. Linus Pauling in 1949, which for the first time linked the specific genetic mutation in patients with sickle cell disease to a demonstrated change in an individual protein, the hemoglobin in the erythrocytes of heterozygous or homozygous individuals.

The Encounter between Biochemistry and Genetics

The development of molecular biology is also the encounter of two disciplines which made considerable progress in the course of the first thirty years of the twentieth century: biochemistry and genetics. The first studies the structure and function of the molecules which make up living things. Between 1900 and 1940, the central processes of metabolism were described: the process of digestion and the absorption of the nutritive elements derived from alimentation, such as the sugars. Every one of these processes is catalysed by a particular enzyme. Enzymes are proteins, like the antibodies present in blood or the proteins responsible for muscular contraction. As a consequence, the study of proteins, of their structure and synthesis, became one of the principal objectives of biochemists.

The second discipline of biology which developed at the beginning of the 20th century is genetics. After the rediscovery of the laws of Mendel through the studies of Hugo de Vries, Carl Correns and Erich von Tschermak in 1900, this science began to take shape thanks to the adoption by Thomas Hunt Morgan, in 1910, of a model organism for genetic studies, the famous fruit fly (Drosophila melanogaster). Shortly after, Morgan showed that the genes are localized on chromosomes. Following this discovery, he continued working with Drosophila and, along with numerous other research groups, confirmed the importance of the gene in the life and development of organisms. Nevertheless, the chemical nature of genes and their mechanisms of action remained a mystery. Molecular biologists committed themselves to the determination of the structure, and the description of the complex relations between, genes and proteins.

The development of molecular biology was not just the fruit of some sort of intrinsic "necessity" in the history of ideas, but was a characteristically historical phenomenon, with all of its unknowns, imponderables and contingencies: the remarkable developments in physics at the beginning of the 20th century highlighted the relative lateness in development in biology, which became the "new frontier" in the search for knowledge about the empirical world. Moreover, the developments of the theory of information and cybernetics in the 1940s, in response to military exigencies, brought to the new biology a significant number of fertile ideas and, especially, metaphors.

The choice of bacteria and of its virus, the bacteriophage, as models for the study of the fundamental mechanisms of life was almost natural - they are the smallest living organisms known to exist - and at the same time the fruit of individual choices. This model owes its success, above all, to the fame and the sense of organization of Max Delbruck, a German physicist, who was able to create a dynamic research group, based in the United States, whose exclusive scope was the study of the bacteriophage: the *School of the Phage*.

The geographic panorama of the developments of the new biology was conditioned above all by preceding work. The US, where genetics had developed the most rapidly, and the UK, where there was a coexistence of both genetics and biochemical research of highly advanced levels, were in the avant-garde. Germany, the cradle of the revolutions in physics, with the best minds and the most advanced laboratories of genetics in the world, should have had a primary role in the development of molecular biology. But history decided differently: the arrival of the Nazis in 1933 - and, to a less extreme degree, the rigidification of totalitarian measures in fascist Italy - caused the emigration of a large number of Jewish and non-Jewish scientists. The majority of them fled to the US or the UK, providing an extra impulse to the scientific dynamism of those nations. These movements ultimately made molecular biology a truly international science from the very beginnings.

History of DNA Biochemistry

The study of DNA is a central part of molecular biology.

First Isolation of DNA

Working in the 19th century, biochemists initially isolated DNA and RNA (mixed together) from cell nuclei. They were relatively quick to appreciate the polymeric nature of their "nucleic acid" isolates, but realized only later that nucleotides were of two types—one containing ribose and the other deoxyribose. It was this subsequent discovery that led to the identification and naming of DNA as a substance distinct from RNA.

Friedrich Miescher (1844–1895) discovered a substance he called "nuclein" in 1869. Somewhat later, he isolated a pure sample of the material now known as DNA from the sperm of salmon, and in 1889 his pupil, Richard Altmann, named it "nucleic acid". This substance was found to exist only in the chromosomes.

In 1919 Phoebus Levene at the Rockefeller Institute identified the components (the four bases, the sugar and the phosphate chain) and he showed that the components of DNA were linked in the order phosphate-sugar-base. He called each of these units a nucleotide and suggested the DNA molecule consisted of a string of nucleotide units linked together through the phosphate groups, which are the 'backbone' of the molecule. However Levene thought the chain was short and that the bases repeated in the same fixed order. Torbjorn Caspersson and Einar Hammersten showed that DNA was a polymer.

Chromosomes and Inherited Traits

Max Delbruck, Nikolai V. Timofeeff-Ressovsky, and Karl G. Zimmer published results in 1935 suggesting that chromosomes are very large molecules the structure of which can be changed by treatment with X-rays, and that by so changing their structure it was possible to change the heritable characteristics governed by those chromosomes. In 1937 William Astbury produced the first X-ray diffraction patterns from DNA. He was not able to propose the correct structure but the patterns showed that DNA had a regular structure and therefore it might be possible to deduce what this structure was.

In 1943, Oswald Theodore Avery and a team of scientists discovered that traits proper to the "smooth" form of the *Pneumococcus* could be transferred to the "rough" form of the same bacteria merely by making the killed "smooth" (S) form available to the live "rough" (R) form. Quite unexpectedly, the living R *Pneumococcus* bacteria were transformed into a new strain of the S form, and the transferred S characteristics turned out to be heritable. Avery called the medium of transfer of traits the transforming principle; he identified DNA as the transforming principle, and not protein as previously thought. He essentially redid Frederick Griffith's experiment. In 1953, Alfred Hershey and Martha Chase did an experiment (Hershey-Chase experiment) that showed, in T2 phage, that DNA is the genetic material (Hershey shared the Nobel prize with Luria).

Discovery of the Structure of DNA

In the 1950s, three groups made it their goal to determine the structure of DNA. The first group to start was at King's College

London and was led by Maurice Wilkins and was later joined by Rosalind Franklin. Another group consisting of Francis Crick and James D. Watson was at Cambridge. A third group was at Caltech and was led by Linus Pauling. Crick and Watson built physical models using metal rods and balls, in which they incorporated the known chemical structures of the nucleotides, as well as the known position of the linkages joining one nucleotide to the next along the polymer. At King's College Maurice Wilkins and Rosalind Franklin examined X-ray diffraction patterns of DNA fibres. Of the three groups, only the London group was able to produce good quality diffraction patterns and thus produce sufficient quantitative data about the structure.

Helix Structure

In 1948 Pauling discovered that many proteins included helical shapes. Pauling had deduced this structure from X-ray patterns and from attempts to physically model the structures. (Pauling was also later to suggest an incorrect three chain helical DNA structure based on Astbury's data.) Even in the initial diffraction data from DNA by Maurice Wilkins, it was evident that the structure involved helices. But this insight was only a beginning. There remained the questions of how many strands came together, whether this number was the same for every helix, whether the bases pointed toward the helical axis or away, and ultimately what were the explicit angles and coordinates of all the bonds and atoms. Such questions motivated the modelling efforts of Watson and Crick.

Complementary Nucleotides

In their modelling, Watson and Crick restricted themselves to what they saw as chemically and biologically reasonable. Still, the breadth of possibilities was very wide. A breakthrough occurred in 1952, when Erwin Chargaff visited Cambridge and inspired Crick with a description of experiments Chargaff had published in 1947. Chargaff had observed that the proportions of the four nucleotides vary between one DNA sample and the next, but that for particular pairs of nucleotides — adenine and thymine, guanine and cytosine — the two nucleotides are always present in equal proportions. Using X-ray diffraction, as well as other data from Rosalind Franklin and her information that the bases were paired, James D. Watson and Francis Crick arrived at the first accurate model of DNA's molecular structure in 1953, which was accepted through inspection by Rosalind Franklin.

The discovery was made on February 28, 1953; the first Watson/ Crick paper appeared in Nature on April 25, 1953. Sir Lawrence Bragg, the director of the Cavendish Laboratory, where Watson and Crick worked, gave a talk at Guys Hospital Medical School in London on Thursday, May 14, 1953 which resulted in an article by Ritchie Calder in The News Chronicle of London, on Friday, May 15, 1953, entitled "Why You Are You. Nearer Secret of Life." The news reached readers of The New York Times the next day; Victor K. McElheny, in researching his biography, "Watson and DNA: Making a Scientific Revolution", found a clipping of a six-paragraph New York Times article written from London and dated May 16, 1953 with the headline "Form of `Life Unit' in Cell Is Scanned." The article ran in an early edition and was then pulled to make space for news deemed more important.(The New York Times subsequently ran a longer article on June 12, 1953). The Cambridge University undergraduate newspaper also ran its own short article on the discovery on Saturday, May 30, 1953. Bragg's original announcement at a Solvay conference on proteins in Belgium on 8 April 1953 went unreported by the press! In 1962 Watson, Crick, and Maurice Wilkins jointly received the Nobel Prize for Physiology or Medicine for their determination of the structure of DNA.

"Central Dogma"

Watson and Crick's model attracted great interest immediately upon its presentation. Arriving at their conclusion on February 21, 1953, Watson and Crick made their first announcement on February 28. In an influential presentation in 1957, Crick laid out the "Central Dogma", which foretold the relationship between DNA, RNA, and proteins, and articulated the "sequence hypothesis." A critical confirmation of the replication mechanism that was implied by the double-helical structure followed in 1958 in the form of the Meselson-Stahl experiment. Work by Crick and coworkers showed that the genetic code was based on non-overlapping triplets of bases, called codons, and Har Gobind Khorana and others deciphered the genetic code not long afterward (1966). These findings represent the birth of molecular biology.

History of RNA Tertiary Structure

Pre-history : The Helical Structure of RNA

The earliest work in RNA structural biology coincided, more or less, with the work being done on DNA in the early 1950s. In their seminal 1953 paper, Watson and Crick suggested that van der Waals crowding by the 2'OH group of ribose would preclude RNA from adopting a double helical structure identical to the model they proposed - what we now know as B-form DNA. This provoked questions about the three dimensional structure of RNA: could this molecule form some type of helical structure, and if so, how? As with DNA, early structural work on RNA centered around isolation of native RNA polymers for fibre diffraction analysis. In part because of heterogeneity of the samples tested, early fibre diffraction patterns were usually ambiguous and not readily interpretable. In 1955, Grunberg-Manago *et al.* published a paper describing the enzyme polynucleotide phosphorylase, which cleaved a phosphate group from nucleotide diphosphates to catalyse their polymerization. This discovery allowed researchers to synthesize homogenous nucleotide polymers, which they then combined to produce double stranded molecules. These samples yielded the most readily interpretable fibre diffraction patterns yet obtained, suggesting an ordered, helical structure for cognate, double stranded RNA that differed from that observed in DNA. These results paved the way for a series of investigations into the various properties and propensities of RNA. Through the late 1950s and early 1960s, numerous papers were publihed on various topics in RNA structure, including RNA-DNA hybridization, triple stranded RNA, and even small-scale crystallography of RNA di-nucleotides - G-C, and A-U - in primitive helix-like arrangements. For a more in-depth review of the early work in RNA structural biology.

The Beginning: Crystal Structure of tRNA

In the mid-1960s, the role of tRNA in protein synthesis was being intensively studied. At this point, ribosomes had been implicated in protein synthesis, and it had been shown that an mRNA strand was necessary for the formation of these structures. In a 1964 publication, Warner and Rich showed that ribosomes active in protein synthesis contained tRNA molecules bound at the A and P sites, and discussed the notion that these molecules aided in the peptidyl transferase reaction. However, despite considerable biochemical characterization, the structural basis of tRNA function remained a mystery. In 1965, Holley *et al.* purified and sequenced the first tRNA molecule, initially proposing that it adopted a cloverleaf structure, based largely on the ability of certain regions of the molecule to form stem loop structures. The isolation of tRNA proved to be the first major windfall in RNA structural biology. Following Holley's publication, numerous investigators began work on isolation tRNA for crystallographic study, developing improved methods for isolating the molecule as they worked.

By 1968 several groups had produced tRNA crystals, but these proved to be of limited quality and did not yield data at the resolutions necessary to determine structure. In 1971, Kim *et al.* achieved another breakthrough, producing crystals of yeast tRNA that diffracted to 2-3 Angstrom resolutions by using spermine, a naturally occurring polyamine, which bound to and stabilized the tRNA. Despite having suitable crystals, however, the structure of tRNA was not immediately solved at high resolution; rather it took pioneering work in the use of heavy metal derivatives and a good deal more time to produce a high-quality density map of the entire molecule. In 1973, Kim *et al.* produced a 4 Angstrom map of the tRNA molecule in which they could unambiguously trace the entire backbone. This solution would be followed by many more, as various investigators worked to refine the structure and thereby more thoroughly elucidate the details of base pairing and stacking interactions, and validate the published architecture of the molecule.

The tRNA structure is notable in the field of nucleic acid structure in general, as it represented the first solution of a long-chain nucleic acid structure of any kind - RNA or DNA - preceding Dickerson's solution of a B-form dodecamer by nearly a decade. Also, tRNA demonstrated many of the tertiary interactions observed in RNA architecture which would not be categorized and more thoroughly understood for years to come, providing a foundation for all future RNA structural research.

The Renaissance: The Hammerhead Ribozyme and the Group I Intron: $P_{4\text{-}6}$

For a considerable time following the first tRNA structures, the field of RNA structure did not dramatically advance. The ability to study an RNA strcuture depended upon the potential to isolate the RNA target. This proved limiting to the field for many years, in part owing to the fact that other know targets - i.e. the ribosome - were significantly more difficult to isolate and crystallize. Further, because other interesting RNA targets had simply not been identified, or were not sufficiently understood to be deemed interesting, there was simply a lack of things to study structurally. As such, for some twenty years following the original publication of the tRNA structure, the structures of only a handful of other RNA targets were solved, with almost all of these belonging to the transfer RNA family. This unfortunate lack of scope would eventually be overcome largely because of two major advancements in nucleic acid research: the identification of ribozymes, and the ability to produce them via *in vitro* transcription.

Subsequent to Tom Cech's publication implicating the *Tetrahymena* group I intron as an autocatalytic ribozyme, and Sidney Altman's report of catalysis by ribonuclease P RNA, several other catalytic RNAs were identified in the late 1980s, including the hammerhead ribozyme. In 1994, McKay *et al.* published the structure of a 'hammerhead RNA-DNA ribozyme-inhibitor complex' at 2.6 Angstrom resolution, in which the autocatalytic activity of the ribozyme was disrupted via binding to a DNA substrate. The conformation of the ribozyme published in this paper was eventually shown to be one of several possible states, and although this particular sample was catalytically inactive, subsequent structures have revealed its active-state architecture. This structure was followed by Doudna's publication of the structure of the P4-P6 domains of the *Tetrahymena* group I intron, a fragment of the ribozyme originally made famous by Cech. The second clause in the title of this publication - *Principles of RNA Packing* - concisely evinces the value of these two structures: for the first time, comparisons could be made between well described tRNA structures and those of globular RNAs outside the transfer family. This allowed the framework of categorization to be built for RNA tertiary structure. It was now possible to propose the conservation of motifs, folds, and various local stabilizing interactions. For an early review of these structures and their implications.

In addition to the advances being made in global structure determination via crystallography, the early 1990s also saw the implementation of NMR as a powerful technique in RNA structural biology. Coincident with the large-scale ribozyme structures being solved crystallographically, a number of structures of small RNAs and RNAs complexed with drugs and peptides were solved using NMR. In addition, NMR was now being used to investigate and supplement crystal structures, as exemplified by the determination of an isolated tetraloop-receptor motif structure published in 1997. Investigations such as this enabled a more precise characterization of the base pairing and base stacking interactions which stabilized the global folds of large RNA molecules. The importance of understanding RNA tertiary structural motifs was prophetically well described by Michel and Costa in their publication identifying the tetraloop motif: "..it should not come as a surprise if self-folding RNA molecules were to make intensive use of only a relatively small set of tertiary motifs. Identifying these motifs would greatly aid modelling enterprises, which will remain essential as long as the crystallization of large RNAs remains a difficult task".

The Modern Era: The Age of RNA Structural Biology

The resurgence of RNA structural biology in the mid-1990s has caused a veritable explosion in the field of nucleic acid structural research. Since the publication of the hammerhead and P_{4-6} structures, numerous major contributions to the field have been made. Some of the most noteworthy examples include the structures of the Group I and Group II introns, and the Ribosome. It should be noted that the first three structures were produced using *in vitro* transcription, and that NMR has played a role in investigating partial components of all four structures - testaments to the indispensability of both techniques for RNA research. Most recently, the 2009 Nobel Prize in Chemistry was awarded to Ada Yonath, Venkatraman Ramakrishnan, and Thomas Steitz for their structural work on the ribosome, demonstrating the prominent role RNA structural biology has taken in modern molecular biology.

History of Protein Biochemistry

First Isolation and Classification

Proteins were recognized as a distinct class of biological molecules in the eighteenth century by Antoine Fourcroy and others. Members of this class (called the "albuminoids", *Eiweisskorper*, or *matières albuminoides*) were recognized by their ability to coagulate or flocculate under various treatments such as heat or acid; well-known examples at the start of the nineteenth century included albumen from egg whites, blood serum albumin, fibrin, and wheat gluten. The similarity between the cooking of egg whites and the curdling of milk was recognized even in ancient times; for example, the name *albumen* for the egg-white protein was coined by Pliny the Elder from the Latin *albus ovi* (egg white).

With the advice of Jons Jakob Berzelius, the Dutch chemist Gerhardus Johannes Mulder carried out elemental analyses of common animal and plant proteins. To everyone's surprise, all proteins had nearly the same empirical formula, roughly $C_{400}H_{620}N_{100}O_{120}$ with individual sulfur and phosphorus atoms. Mulder published his findings in two papers (1837,1838) and hypothesized that there was one basic substance (*Grundstoff*) of proteins, and that it was synthesized by plants and absorbed from them by animals in digestion. Berzelius was an early proponent of this theory and proposed the name "protein" for this substance in a letter dated 10 July 1838

Mulder went on to identify the products of protein degradation such as the amino acid, leucine, for which he found a (nearly correct) molecular weight of 131 Da.

Purifications and Measurements of Mass

The minimum molecular weight suggested by Mulder's analyses was roughly 9 kDa, hundreds of times larger than other molecules being studied. Hence, the chemical structure of proteins (their primary structure) was an active area of research until 1949, when Fred Sanger sequenced insulin. The (correct) theory that proteins were linear polymers of amino acids linked by peptide bonds was proposed independently and simultaneously by Franz Hofmeister and Emil Fischer at the same conference in 1902. However, some scientists were sceptical that such long macromolecules could be stable in solution. Consequently, numerous alternative theories of the protein primary structure were proposed, e.g., the colloidal hypothesis that proteins were assemblies of small molecules, the cyclol hypothesis of Dorothy Wrinch, the diketopiperazine hypothesis of Emil Abderhalden and the pyrrol/piperidine hypothesis of Troensgard (1942). Most of these theories had difficulties in accounting for the fact that the digestion of proteins yielded peptides and amino acids. Proteins were finally shown to be macromolecules of well-defined composition (and not colloidal mixtures) by Theodor Svedberg using analytical ultracentrifugation. The possibility that some proteins are non-covalent associations of such macromolecules was shown by Gilbert Smithson Adair (by measuring the osmotic pressure of hemoglobin) and, later, by Frederic M. Richards in his studies of ribonuclease S. The mass spectrometry of proteins has long been a useful technique for identifying posttranslational modifications and, more recently, for probing protein structure.

Most proteins are difficult to purify in more than milligram quantities, even using the most modern methods. Hence, early studies focused on proteins that could be purified in large quantities, e.g., those of blood, egg white, various toxins, and digestive/metabolic enzymes obtained from slaughterhouses. Many techniques of protein purification were developed during World War II in a project led by Edwin Joseph Cohn to purify blood proteins to help keep soldiers alive. In the late 1950s, the Armour Hot Dog Co. purified 1 kg (= one million milligrams) of pure bovine pancreatic ribonuclease A and made it freely available to scientists around the world. This generous act made RNase A the main protein for basic research for the next few decades, resulting in several Nobel Prizes.

Protein Folding and First Structural Models

The study of protein folding began in 1910 with a famous paper by Henrietta Chick and C. J. Martin, in which they showed that the flocculation of a protein was composed of two distinct processes: the precipitation of a protein from solution was *preceded* by another process called denaturation, in which the protein became much less soluble, lost its enzymatic activity and became more chemically reactive. In the mid-1920s, Tim Anson and Alfred Mirsky proposed that denaturation was a reversible process, a correct hypothesis that was initially lampooned by some scientists as "unboiling the egg". Anson also suggested that denaturation was a two-state ("all-or-none") process, in which one fundamental molecular transition resulted in the drastic changes in solubility, enzymatic activity and chemical reactivity; he further noted that the free energy changes upon denaturation were much smaller than those typically involved in chemical reactions.

In 1929, Hsien Wu hypothesized that denaturation was protein unfolding, a purely conformational change that resulted in the exposure of amino acid side chains to the solvent. According to this (correct) hypothesis, exposure of aliphatic and reactive side chains to solvent rendered the protein less soluble and more reactive, whereas the loss of a specific conformation caused the loss of enzymatic activity. Although considered plausible, Wu's hypothesis was not immediately accepted, since so little was known of protein structure and enzymology and other factors could account for the changes in solubility, enzymatic activity and chemical reactivity. In the early 1960s, Chris Anfinsen showed that the folding of ribonuclease A was fully reversible with no external cofactors needed, verifying the "thermodynamic hypothesis" of protein folding that the folded state represents the global minimum of free energy for the protein.

The hypothesis of protein folding was followed by research into the physical interactions that stabilize folded protein structures. The crucial role of hydrophobic interactions was hypothesized by Dorothy Wrinch and Irving Langmuir, as a mechanism that might stabilize her cyclol structures. Although supported by J. D. Bernal and others, this (correct) hypothesis was rejected along with the cyclol hypothesis, which was disproven in the 1930s by Linus Pauling (among others). Instead, Pauling championed the idea that protein structure was stabilized mainly by hydrogen bonds, an idea advanced initially by William Astbury (1933). Remarkably, Pauling's incorrect theory about H-bonds resulted in his *correct* models for the secondary structure elements of proteins, the alpha helix and the beta sheet. The hydrophobic interaction was restored to its correct prominence by a famous article in 1959 by Walter Kauzmann on denaturation, based partly on work by Kaj Linderstrom-Lang. The ionic nature of proteins was demonstrated by Bjerrum, Weber and Arne Tiselius, but Linderstrom-Lang showed that the charges were generally accessible to solvent and not bound to each other (1949).

The secondary and low-resolution tertiary structure of globular proteins was investigated initially by hydrodynamic methods, such as analytical ultracentrifugation and flow birefringence. Spectroscopic methods to probe protein structure (such as circular dichroism, fluorescence, near-ultraviolet and infrared absorbance) were developed in the 1950s. The first atomic-resolution structures of proteins were solved by X-ray crystallography in the 1960s and by NMR in the 1980s. As of 2006, the Protein Data Bank has nearly 40,000 atomic-resolution structures of proteins. In more recent times, cryo-electron microscopy of large macromolecular assemblies and computational protein structure prediction of small protein domains are two methods approaching atomic resolution.

RNA

Ribonucleic acid (RNA) is one of the three major macromolecules (along ith DNA and proteins) that are essential for all known forms of life.

Like DNA, RNA is made up of a long chain of components called nucleotides. Each nucleotide consists of a nucleobase (sometimes called a nitrogenous base), a ribose sugar, and a phosphategroup. The sequence of nucleotides allows RNA to encode genetic information. For example, someviruses use RNA instead of DNA as their genetic material, and all organisms use messenger RNA(mRNA) to carry the genetic information that directs the synthesis of proteins.

Like proteins, some RNA molecules play an active role in cells by catalyzing biological reactions, controlling gene expression, or sensing and communicating responses to cellular signals. One of these active processes is protein synthesis, a universal function whereby mRNA molecules direct the assembly of proteins on ribosomes. This process uses transfer RNA (tRNA) molecules to deliver amino acids to the ribosome, where ribosomal RNA (rRNA) links amino acids together to form proteins.

The chemical structure of RNA is very similar to that of DNA, with two differences—(a) RNA contains the sugar ribose while DNA contains the slightly different sugar deoxyribose (a type of ribose that lacks one oxygen atom), and (b) RNA has the nucleobase uracil while DNA contains thymine (uracil and thymine have similar base-pairing properties).

Unlike DNA, most RNA molecules are single-stranded. Single-stranded RNA molecules adopt very complex three-dimensional structures, since they are not restricted to the repetitive double-helical form of double-stranded DNA. RNA is made within living cells by RNA polymerases, enzymes which act to copy a DNA or RNA template into a new RNA strand through processes known as transcriptionor RNA replication, respectively.

Comparison with DNA

RNA and DNA are both nucleic acids, but differ in three main ways. First, unlike DNA which is generally double-stranded, RNA is a single-stranded molecule in many of its biological roles and has a much shorter chain of nucleotides. Second, while DNA contains *deoxyribose*, RNA contains *ribose* (there is no hydroxyl group attached to the pentose ring in the 2' position in DNA). These hydroxyl groups make RNA less stable than DNA because it is more prone to hydrolysis. Third, the complementary base to adenine is not thymine, as it is in DNA, but rather uracil, which is anunmethylated form of thymine.

Like DNA, most biologically active RNAs, including mRNA, tRNA, rRNA, snRNAs and other non-coding RNAs, contain self-complementary sequences that allow parts of the RNA to fold and pair with itself to form double helices. Structural analysis of these RNAs has revealed that they are highly structured. Unlike DNA, their structures do not consist of long double helices but rather collections of short helices packed together into structures akin to proteins. In this fashion, RNAs can achieve chemical catalysis, like enzymes. For instance, determination of the structure of the ribosome—an enzyme that catalyses peptide bond formation—revealed that its active site is composed entirely of RNA.

Structure

Each nucleotide in RNA contains a ribose sugar, with carbons numbered 1' through 5'. A base is attached to the 1' position, generally adenine (A), cytosine (C), guanine (G) or uracil (U). Adenine and guanine are purines, cytosine and uracil are pyrimidines. A phosphate group is attached to the 3' position of one ribose and the 5' position of the next. The phosphate groups have a negative charge each at physiological pH, making RNA a charged molecule (polyanion). The bases may form hydrogen bonds between cytosine and guanine, between adenine and uracil and between guanine and uracil. However other interactions are possible, such as a group of adenine bases binding to each other in a bulge, or the GNRA tetraloop that has a guanine–adenine base-pair.n important structural feature of RNA that distinguishes it from DNA is the presence of ahydroxyl group at the 2' position of the ribose sugar. The presence of this functional group causes the helix to adopt the A-form geometry rather than the B-form most commonly observed in DNA. This results in a very deep and narrow major groove and a shallow and wide minor groove. A second consequence of the presence of the 2'-hydroxyl group is that in conformationally flexible regions of an RNA molecule (that is, not involved in formation of a double helix), it can chemically attack the adjacent phosphodiester bond to cleave the backbone. RNA is transcribed with only four bases (adenine, cytosine, guanine and uracil), but these bases and attached sugars can be modified in numerous ways as the RNAs mature. Pseudouridine (y), in which the linkage between uracil and ribose is changed from a C–N bond to a C–C bond, and ribothymidine (T), are found in various places (most notably in the TyC loop of tRNA). Another notable modified base is hypoxanthine, a deaminated adenine base whose nucleoside is called inosine (I). Inosine plays a key role in the wobble hypothesis of thegenetic code.

There are nearly 100 other naturally occurring modified nucleosides, of which pseudouridine and nucleosides with 2'-O-methylribose are the most common. The specific roles of many of these modifications in RNA are not fully understood. However, it is notable that in ribosomal RNA, many of the post-transcriptional modifications occur in highly functional regions, such as the peptidyl transferase centre and the subunit interface, implying that they are important for normal function.

The functional form of single stranded RNA molecules, just like proteins, frequently requires a specific tertiary structure. The scaffold for this structure is provided by secondary structural elements which are hydrogen bonds within the molecule. This leads to several recognizable “domains” of secondary structure like hairpin loops, bulges and internal loops. Since RNA is charged, metal ions such as Mg^{2+} are needed to stabilise many secondary and tertiary structures.

Synthesis

Synthesis of RNA is usually catalysed by an enzyme—RNA polymerase—using DNA as a template, a process known as transcription. Initiation of transcription begins with the binding of the enzyme to a promoter sequence in the DNA (usually found "upstream" of a gene). The DNA double helix is unwound by the helicase activity of the enzyme. The enzyme then progresses along the template strand in the 3' to 5' direction, synthesizing a complementary RNA molecule with elongation occurring in the 5' to 3' direction. The DNA sequence also dictates where termination of RNA synthesis will occur.

RNAs are often modified by enzymes after transcription. For example, a poly(A) tail and a 5' cap are added to eukaryotic pre-mRNA andintrons are removed by the spliceosome.

There are also a number of RNA-dependent RNA polymerases that use RNA as their template for synthesis of a new strand of RNA. For instance, a number of RNA viruses (such as poliovirus) use this type of enzyme to replicate their genetic material. Also, RNA-dependent RNA polymerase is part of the RNA interference pathway in many organisms.

Messenger RNA

Messenger RNA (mRNA) is a molecule of RNA encoding a chemical "blueprint" for a protein product. mRNA is transcribed from a DNA template, and carries coding information to the sites of protein synthesis: the ribosomes. Here, the nucleic acid polymer is translated into a polymer of amino acids: a protein. In mRNA as in DNA, genetic information is encoded in the sequence of nucleotides arranged into codonsconsisting of three bases each. Each codon encodes for a specific amino acid, except the stop codons that terminate protein synthesis. This process requires two other types of RNA: transfer RNA (tRNA) mediates recognition of the codon and provides the corresponding amino acid, while ribosomal RNA (rRNA) is the central component of the ribosome's protein manufacturing machinery.

Synthesis, Processing, and Function

The brief existence of an mRNA molecule begins with transcription and ultimately ends in degradation. During its life, an mRNA molecule may also be processed, edited, and transported prior to translation. Eukaryotic mRNA molecules often require extensive processing and transport, while prokaryotic molecules do not.

Transcription

During transcription, RNA polymerase makes a copy of a gene from the DNA to mRNA as needed. This process is similar in eukaryotes and prokaryotes. One notable difference, however, is that prokaryotic

RNA polymerase associates with mRNA processing enzymes during transcription so that processing can proceed quickly after the start of transcription. The short-lived, unprocessed or partially processed, product is termed *pre-mRNA*; once completely processed, it is termed *mature mRNA*.

Eukaryotic Pre-mRNA Processing

Processing of mRNA differs greatly among eukaryotes, bacteria and archea. Non-eukaryotic mRNA is essentially mature upon transcription and requires no processing, except in rare cases. Eukaryotic pre-mRNA, however, requires extensive processing.

5' Cap Addition

A *5' cap* (also termed an RNA cap, an RNA 7-methylguanosine cap or an RNA m^7G cap) is a modified guanine nucleotide that has been added to the "front" or 5' end of a eukaryotic messenger RNA shortly after the start of transcription. The 5' cap consists of a terminal 7-methylguanosine residue which is linked through a 5'-5'-triphosphate bond to the first transcribed nucleotide. Its presence is critical for recognition by the ribosome and protection from RNases.

Cap addition is coupled to transcription, and occurs co-transcriptionally, such that each influences the other. Shortly after the start of transcription, the 5' end of the mRNA being synthesized is bound by a cap-synthesizing complex associated with RNA polymerase. Thisenzymatic complex catalyses the chemical reactions that are required for mRNA capping. Synthesis proceeds as a multi-step biochemicalreaction.

Splicing

Splicing is the process by which pre-mRNA is modified to remove certain stretches of non-coding sequences called introns; the stretches that remain include protein-coding sequences and are called exons. Sometimes pre-mRNA messages may be spliced in several different ways, allowing a single gene to encode multiple proteins. This process is called alternative splicing. Splicing is usually performed by an RNA-protein complex called the spliceosome, but some RNA molecules are also capable of catalyzing their own splicing.

Editing

In some instances, an mRNA will be edited, changing the nucleotide composition of that mRNA. An example in humans is the apolipoprotein B mRNA, which is edited in some tissues, but not others. The editing creates an early stop codon, which upon translation, produces a shorter protein.

Polyadenylation

Polyadenylation is the covalent linkage of a polyadenylyl moiety to a messenger RNA molecule. In eukaryotic organisms, most messenger RNA (mRNA) molecules are polyadenylated at the 3' end. The poly(A) tail and the protein bound to it aid in protecting mRNA from degradation by exonucleases. Polyadenylation is also important for transcription termination, export of the mRNA from the nucleus, and translation. mRNA can also be polyadenylated in prokaryotic organisms, where poly(A) tails act to facilitate, rather than impede, exonucleolytic degradation.

Polyadenylation occurs during and immediately after transcription of DNA into RNA. After transcription has been terminated, the mRNA chain is cleaved through the action of an endonuclease complex associated with RNA polymerase. After the mRNA has been cleaved, around 250 adenosine residues are added to the free 3' end at the cleavage site. This reaction is catalysed by polyadenylate polymerase. Just as in alternative splicing, there can be more than one polyadenylation variant of a mRNA.

Transport

Another difference between eukaryotes and prokaryotes is mRNA transport. Because eukaryotic transcription and translation is compartmentally separated, eukaryotic mRNAs must be exported from the nucleus to the cytoplasm. Mature mRNAs are recognized by their processed modifications and then exported through the nuclear pore. In neurons mRNA must be transported from the soma to the dendriteswhere local translation occurs in response to external stimuli. Many messages are marked with so-called "zip codes" which targets their transport to a specific location.

Translation

Because prokaryotic mRNA does not need to be processed or transported, translation by the ribosome can begin immediately after the end of transcription. Therefore, it can be said that prokaryotic translation is *coupled* to transcription and occurs *co-transcriptionally*. Eukaryotic mRNA that has been processed and transported to the cytoplasm (i.e. mature mRNA) can then be translated by the ribosome. Translation may occur at ribosomes free-floating in the cytoplasm, or directed to the endoplasmic reticulum by the signal recognition particle. Therefore, unlike prokaryotes, eukaryotic translation *is not* directly coupled to transcription.

5' cap

The 5' cap is a specially altered nucleotide on the 5' end of precursor messenger RNA and some other primary RNA transcripts as found ineukaryotes and, as a special exception, caliciviruses such as noroviruses. The process of 5' capping is vital to creating mature messenger RNA, which is then able to undergo translation. Capping ensures the messenger RNA's stability while it undergoes translation in the process of protein synthesis, and is a highly regulated process that occurs in the cell nucleus.

5' Cap Structure

The 5' cap is found on the 5' end of an mRNA molecule and consists of a guanine nucleotide connected to the mRNA via an unusual 5' to 5' triphosphate linkage. This guanosine is methylated on the 7 position directly after capping *in vitro* by a methyl transferase. It is referred to as a 7-methylguanosine cap, abbreviated m^7G.

Further modifications include the possible methylation of the 2' hydroxy-groups of the first 3 ribose sugars of the 5' end of the mRNA. The methylation of both 2' hydroxy-groups is shown on the diagram.

The 5' cap looks like the 3' end of an RNA molecule (the 5' carbon of the cap ribose is bonded, and the 3' unbonded). This provides significant resistance to 5' exonucleases.

Capping Process

The starting point is the unaltered 5' end of an RNA molecule. This features a final nucleotide followed by three phosphate groups attached to the 5' carbon.

1. One of the terminal phosphate groups is removed (by a phosphatase), leaving two terminal phosphates.
2. GTP is added to the terminal phosphates (by a guanylyl transferase), losing two phosphate groups (from the GTP) in the process. This results in the 5' to 5' triphosphate linkage.
3. The 7-Nitrogen of guanine is methylated (by a methyl transferase).
4. Other methyltransferases are optionally used to carry out methylation of 5' proximal nucleotides.

5' Capping Targeting

The Capping Enzyme Complex (CEC) required for capping is found bound to the RNA polymerase II before transcription starts. As soon as the 5' end of the new transcript emerges the enzymes transfer to it and begin the capping process (this is a similar kind of mechanism to ensure capping as for polyadenylation).

The enzymes for capping can only bind to RNA polymerase II ensuring specificity to only these transcripts, which are almost entirely mRNA.

5' Cap Function

The 5' cap has 4 main functions:

1. Regulation of nuclear export.
2. Prevention of degradation by exonucleases.
3. Promotion of translation.
4. Promotion of 5' proximal intron excision.

Nuclear export of RNA is regulated by the Cap binding complex (CBC), which binds exclusively to capped RNA. The CBC is then recognized by the nuclear pore complex and exported. Once in the cytoplasm after the pioneer round of translation, the CBC complex is replaced by the translation factors eIF-4E and eIF-4G. This complex is then recognized by other translation initiation machinery including the ribosome. Cap prevents 5' degradation in two ways. First, degradation of the mRNA by 5' exonucleases is prevented (as mentioned above) by functionally looking like a 3' end. Second, the CBC complex and the eIF-4E/eIF-4G block the access of decapping enzymes to the cap. This increases the half-life of the mRNA, essential in eukaryotes as the export process takes significant time.

Decapping of an mRNA is catalysed by the decapping complex made up of at least Dcp1 and Dcp2, which must compete with eIF-4E to bind the cap. Thus the 5' cap is a marker of an actively translating mRNA and is used by cells to regulate mRNA half-lives in response to new stimuli. Undesirable mRNAs are sent to P-bodies for temporary storage or decapping, the details of which are still being resolved.

The mechanism of 5' proximal intron excision promotion is not well understood, but the 5' cap appears to loop around and interact with thespliceosome in the splicing process, promoting intron excision.

Coding Regions

Coding regions are composed of codons, which are decoded and translated (in eukaryotes usually into one and in prokaryotes usually into several) proteins by the ribosome. Coding regions begin with the start codon and end with a stop codon. Generally, the start codon is an AUG triplet and the stop codon is UAA, UAG, or UGA. The coding regions tend to be stabilised by internal base pairs, this impedes degradation. In addition to being protein-coding, portions of coding regions may serve as regulatory sequences in the pre-mRNA asexonic splicing enhancers or exonic splicing silencers. .

Five Prime Untranslated Region

The five prime untranslated region (5' UTR), also known as the leader sequence, is a particular section of messenger RNA (mRNA) and the DNA that codes for it. At times the leader sequence can contain elements for control gene expression by way of attenuation.

The leader sequence will be translated and the availability of the encoded amino acids will affect the transcription of the rest of the mRNA. It starts at the +1 position (where transcription begins) and ends one nucleotide before the start codon (usually AUG) of the coding region. It usually contains a ribosome binding site (RBS), in bacteria also known as the Shine Dalgarno sequence (AGGAGGU). The 5' UTR may be a hundred or more nucleotides long, and the 3' UTR may be even longer (up to several kilobases in length) .

An mRNA molecule codes for a protein through translation. The mRNA also contains regions that are not translated: in eukaryotes this includes the 5' untranslated region, 3' untranslated region, 5' cap and poly-A tail.

In prokaryotic mRNA the 5' UTR is normally short. Some viruses and cellular genes have unusual long structured 5' UTRs which may have roles in gene expression.

Several regulatory sequences may be found in the 5' UTR:

* Binding sites for proteins, that may affect the mRNA's stability or translation, for example iron responsive elements, which occur in the 5' UTRs (and 3' UTRs) of a small number ofeukaryotic mRNAs that regulate gene expression in response to iron.
* Regulatory elements that do not depend on proteins, such asriboswitches.
* Sequences that promote the initiation of translation.

Three Prime Untranslated Region

The three prime untranslated region (3' UTR) is a particular section of messenger RNA (mRNA). It follows the coding region.

An mRNA molecule codes for a protein through translation. The mRNA also contains regions that are not translated. In eukaryotes these regions are the cap, 5' untranslated region, 3' untranslated region, and polyA tail.

In prokaryotes mRNA structures have some differences (seemRNA) as do histone mRNAs. However, both have 3' UTRs.

Several regulatory sequences are found in the 3' UTR:

* A polyadenylation signal, usually *AAUAAA*, or a slight variant. This marks the site of cleavage of the transcript approximately 30 base pairs past the signal, followed by the addition of several hundred adenine residues (poly-A tail).
* Binding sites for proteins, that may affect the mRNA's stability or location in the cell, like SECIS elements (which direct the ribosome to translate the codon UGA as selenocysteines rather than as a stop codon), or AU-rich elements (AREs), stretches consisting of mainlyadenine and uracil nucleotides (which can either stabilize or destabilize the mRNA depending on the protein bound to it).
* Binding sites for miRNAs, a type of RNAi.

Polyadenylation

Polyadenylation is the addition of a poly(A) tail to an RNAmolecule. The poly(A) tail consists of multiple adenosine monophosphates; in other words, it is a stretch of RNA which only has Adenine bases. In eukaryotes, polyadenylation is part of the process that produces mature messenger RNA(mRNA) for translation. It therefore forms part of the larger process of gene expression.

The process of polyadenylation begins as the transcription of a gene finishes. The 3'-most segment of the newly-made RNA is first cleaved off by a set of proteins; these proteins then synthesise the poly(A) tail at the RNA's 3' end. In some genes these proteins may add a poly(A) tail at any one of several possible sites, polyadenylation can therefore produce more than one transcript from a single gene, similar to alternative splicing.

The poly(A) tail is important for the nuclear export, translation and stability of mRNA. The tail is shortened over time and when it is short enough, the mRNA is enzymatically degraded.

However, in a few cell types, mRNAs with short poly(A) tails are stored for later activation by re-polyadenylation in the cytosol. In contrast, when polyadenylation occurs in bacteria, it promotes RNA degradation. This is also sometimes the case for eukaryotic non-coding RNAs. The wide distribution of polyadenylation among living organisms indicates that this process evolved early in the history of life on Earth.

Primer on RNA

RNAs are a type of large biological molecules, whose individual building blocks are called nucleotides. The name *poly(A) tail* (for polyadenylic acid tail) reflects the way RNA nucleotides are abbreviated, with a letter for the base the nucleotide contains (A for adenine, C for cytosine, G for guanine and U for uracil). RNAs are produced (*transcribed*) from a DNA template. By convention, RNA sequences are written in a 5' to 3' direction.

The 5' end is the part of the RNA molecule that is transcribed first, and the 3' end is transcribed last. The 3' end is also where the poly(A) tail is found on polyadenylated RNAs.

Messenger RNA (mRNA) is RNA that has a coding region that acts as a template for protein synthesis (*translation*). The rest of the mRNA, the *untranslated regions*, tune how active the mRNA is. There are also many RNAs that are not translated, called non-coding RNAs. Like the untranslated regions, many of these non-coding RNAs have regulatory roles.

Nuclear Polyadenylation

Function

In nuclear polyadenylation, a poly(A) tail is added to an RNA at the end of transcription. On mRNAs, the poly(A) tail protects the mRNA molecule from enzymatic degradation in the cytoplasm and aids in transcription termination, export of the mRNA from the nucleus, and translation. Almost all eukaryotic mRNAs are polyadenylated, with the exception of animal replication dependent histone mRNAs. These are the only mRNAs in eukaryotes that lack a poly(A) tail, ending instead in a stem-loop structure followed by a purine-rich sequence, termed histone downstream element, that directs where the RNA is cut so that the 3' end of the histone mRNA is formed.

Many eukaryotic non-coding RNAs are always polyadenylated at the end of transcription. There are small RNAs where the poly(A) tail is only seen in intermediary forms and not in the mature RNA as the ends are removed during processing, notably microRNAs. But for manylong noncoding RNAs – a seemingly large group of regulatory RNAs that for example includes the RNA Xist which mediates X chromosome inactivation – a poly(A) tail is part of the mature RNA.

Mechanism

The polyadenylation machinery in the nucleus of eukaryotes works on products of RNA polymerase II, such as precursor mRNA. Here, a multi-protein complex cleaves the 3'-most part of a newly produced RNA and polyadenylates the end produced by this cleavage. The cleavage is catalysed by the enzyme CPSF and occurs 10–30 nucleotides downstream of its binding site.This site is often the sequence AAUAAA on the RNA, but variants of it exist that bind more weakly to CPSF. Two other proteins add specificity to the binding to an RNA: CstF and CFI. CstF binds to a GU-rich region further downstream of CPSF's site.CFI recognises a third site on the RNA (a set of UGUAA sequences in mammals) and can recruit CPSF even if the AAUAAA sequence is missing. The polyadenylation signal – the sequence motif recognised by the RNA cleavage complex – varies between groups of eukaryotes. Most human polyadenylation sites contain the AAUAAA sequence, but this sequence is less common in plants and fungi.

The RNA is cleaved right after transcription, as CstF also binds to RNA polymerase II. Cleavage also involves the protein CFII, unknown how. The cleavage site associated with a polyadenylation signal can vary up to some 50 nucleotides. When the RNA is cleaved, polyadenylation starts, catalysed by polyadenylate polymerase. Polyadenylate polymerase builds the poly(A) tail by adding adenosine monophosphate units from adenosine triphosphate to the RNA, cleaving off pyrophosphate. Another protein, PAB2, binds to the new, short poly(A) tail and increases the affinity of polyadenylate polymerase for the RNA. When the poly(A) tail is approximately 250 nucleotides long the enzyme can no longer bind to CPSF and polyadenylation stops, thus determing the length of the poly(A) tail. CPSF is in contact with RNA polymerase II, allowing it to tell the polymerase to terminate transcription. The polyadenylation machinery is also physically linked to the spliceosome, a complex that removes introns from RNAs.

Downstream Effects

The poly(A) tail acts as the binding site for poly(A)-binding protein. Poly(A)-binding protein promotes export from the nucleus and translation, and inhibits degradation. This protein binds to the poly(A) tail prior to mRNA export from the nucleus and in yeast also recruits poly(A) nuclease, an enzyme that shortens the poly(A) tail and allows the export of the mRNA. Poly(A)-binding protein is exported to the cytoplasm with the RNA. mRNAs that are not exported are degraded by the exosome. Poly(A)-binding protein also can bind to, and thus recruit, several proteins that affect translation, one of these is initiation factor-4G which in turn recruits the 40Sribosomal subunit. However, a poly(A) tail is not required for the translation of all mRNAs.

Deadenylation

In eukaryotic somatic cells, the poly(A) tail of most mRNAs in the cytoplasm gradually get shorter, and mRNAs with shorter poly(A) tail are translated less and degraded sooner. However, it can take many hours before an mRNA is degraded. This deadenylation and degradation process can be accelerated by microRNAs complementary to the 3' untranslated region of an mRNA. In immature egg cells, mRNAs with shortened poly(A) tails are not degraded, but are instead stored without being translated. They are then activated by cytoplasmic polyadenylation after fertilisation, during egg activation.

In animals, poly(A) ribonuclease (PARN) can bind to the 5' cap and remove nucleotides from the poly(A) tail. The level of access to the 5' cap and poly(A) tail is important in controlling how soon the mRNA is degraded. PARN deadenylates less if the RNA is bound by the initiation factors 4E (at the 5' cap) and 4G (at the poly(A) tail), so this is why translation reduces deadenylation. The rate of deadenylation may also be regulated by RNA-binding proteins. Once the poly(A) tail is removed, the decapping complex removes the 5' cap, leading to a degradation of the RNA. Several other enzymes that seem to be involved in deadenylation have been identified in yeast.

Alternative Polyadenylation

Many protein-coding genes have more than one polyadenylation site, so a gene can code for several mRNAs that differ in their 3' end. Since alternative polyadenylation changes the length of the 3' untranslated region, it can change which binding sites for microRNAs the 3' untranslated region contains. MicroRNAs tend to repress translation and promote degradation of the mRNAs they bind to, although there are examples of microRNAs that stabilise transcripts. Alternative polyadenylation can also shorten the coding region, thus making the mRNA code for a different protein, but this is much less common than just shortening the 3' untranslated region.

The choice of poly(A) site depends on the expression of the proteins that take part in polyadenylation. For example, the expression of CstF-64, a subunit of cleavage stimulatory factor (CstF), increases in macrophages in response to lipopolysaccharides (a group of bacterial compounds that trigger an immune response). This results in the selection of weak poly(A) sites and thus shorter transcripts.

This removes regulatory elements in the 3' untranslated regions of mRNAs for defence-related products like lysozyme and TNF-a. These mRNAs then have longer half-lives and produce more of these proteins. RNA-binding proteins other than those in the polyadenylation machinery can also affect whether a polyadenyation site is used, as can DNA methylationnear the polyadenylation signal.

Cytoplasmic Polyadenylation

There is polyadenylation in the cytosol of some animal cell types, namely in the germ line, during early embryogenesis and in post-synapticsites of nerve cells. This lengthens the poly(A) tail of an mRNA with a shortened poly(A) tail, so that the mRNA will be translated.These shortened poly(A) tails are often less than 20 nucleotides, and are lengthened to around 80–150 nucleotides.

In the early mouse embryo, cytoplasmic polyadenylation of maternal RNAs from the egg cell allows the cell to survive and grow even though transcription does not start until the middle of the 2-cell stage (4-cell stage in human). In the brain, cytoplasmic polyadenylation is active during learning and could to play a role in long-term potentiation, which is the strengthening of the signal transmission from a nerve cell to another in response to nerve impulses and is important for learning and memory formation.

Cytoplasmic polyadenylation requires the RNA-binding proteins CPSF and CPEB, and can involve other RNA-binding proteins like Pumilio. Depending on the cell type, the polymerase can be the same type of polyadenylate polymerase (PAP) that is used in the nuclear process, or the cytoplasmic polymerase GLD-2.

Tagging for Degradation in Eukaryotes

For many non-coding RNAs, including tRNA, rRNA, snRNA and snoRNA, polyadenylation is a way of marking the RNA for degradation, in at least yeast. This polyadenylation is done in the nucleus by the TRAMP complex, which adds a tail that is around 40 nucleotides long to the 3' end. The RNA is then degraded by the exosome. Poly(A) tails have also been found on human rRNA fragments, both the form of homopolymeric (A only) and heterpolymeric (mostly A) tails.

In Prokaryotes and Organelles

In many bacteria, both mRNAs and non-coding RNAs can be polyadenylated. This poly(A) tail promotes degradation by the degradosome, which contains two RNA-degrading enzymes: polynucleotide phosphorylase and RNase E. Polynucleotide phosphorylase binds to the 3' end of RNAs and the 3' extension provided by the poly(A) tail allows it to bind to the RNAs whose secondary structure would otherwise block the 3' end. Successive rounds of polyadenylation and degradation of the 3' end by polynucleotide phosphorylase allows the degradosome to overcome these secondary structures. The poly(A) tail can also recruit RNases that cut the RNA in two. These bacterial poly(A) tails are about 30 nucleotides long.

In as different groups as animals and trypanosomes, the mitochondria contain both stabilising and destabilising poly(A) tails. Destabilising polyadenylation targets both mRNA and noncoding RNAs. The poly(A) tails are 43 nucleotides long on average. The stabilising ones start at the stop codon, and without them the stop codon (UAA) is not complete as the genome only encodes the U or UA part. Plant mitochondria only have destabilising polyadenylation, and yeast mitochondria have no polyadenylation at all.

While many bacteria and mitochondria have polyadenylate polymerases, they also have another type of polyadenylation, performed bypolynucleotide phosphorylase itself. This enzyme is found in bacteria, mitochondria, plastids and as a constituent of the archeal exosome (in those archaea that have an exosome). It can synthesise a 3' extension where the vast majority of the bases are adenines. Like in bacteria, polyadenylation by polynucleotide phosphorylase promotes degradation of the RNA in plastids and likely also archaea.

Evolution

Although polyadenylation is seen in almost all organisms, it is not universal. However, the wide distribution of this modification and the fact that it is present in organisms from all three domains of life implies that the last universal common ancestor of all living organisms probably had some form of polyadenylation system. A few organisms do not polyadenylate mRNA, which implies that they have lost their polyadenylation machineries during evolution. Although no examples of eukaryotes that lack polyadenylation are known, mRNAs from the bacterium *Mycoplasma gallisepticum* and the salt-tolerant archaean *Haloferax volcanii* lack this modification.

The most ancient polyadenylating enzyme is polynucleotide phosphorylase. This enzyme is part of both the bacterial degradosome and archaeal exosome, two closely related complexes that recycle RNA into nucleotides. This enzyme degrades RNA by attacking the bond between the 3'-most nucleotides with a phosphate, breaking off a diphosphate nucleotide. This reaction is reversible, and so the enzyme can also extend RNA with more nucleotides. The heteropolymeric tail added by polynucleotide phosphorylase is very rich in adenine. The choice of adenine is most likely the result of higher ADP concentrations than other nucleotides as a result of using ATP as an energy currency, making it more likely to be incorporated in this tail in early lifeforms. It has been suggested that the involvement of adenine-rich tails in RNA degradation prompted the later evolution of polyadenylate polymerases (the enzymes that produce poly(A) tails with no other nucleotides in them).

Polyadenylate polymerases are not as ancient. They have separately evolved in both bacteria and eukaryotes from CCA-adding enzyme, which is the enzyme that completes the 3' ends of tRNAs. Its catalytic domain is homologous to that of other polymerases. Likely, the horizontal transfer of bacterial CCA-adding enzyme to eukaryotes allowed the archaeal-like CCA-adding enzyme to switch function to a poly(A) polymerase. Some lineages, like archaea and cyanobacteria, never evolved a polyadenylate polymerase.

History

Polyadenylation was first identified in 1960 as an enzymatic activity in extracts made from cell nuclei that could polymerise ATP, but not ADP, into polyadenine. Although identified in many types of cells, this activity had no known function until 1971, when poly(A) sequences were found in mRNAs. Initially, the only function of these sequences was thought to be protection of the 3' end of the RNA from nucleases, but later the specific roles of polyadenylation in nuclear export and translation were identified. The polymerases responsible for polyadenylation were first purified and characterized in the 1960s and 1970s, but the large number of accessory proteins that control this process were only discovered in the early 1990s.

Monocistronic Versus Polycistronic mRNA

An mRNA molecule is said to be monocistronic when it contains the genetic information to translate only a single protein. This is the case for most of the eukaryotic mRNAs. On the other hand, polycistronic mRNA carries the information of several genes, which are translated into several proteins. These proteins usually have a related function and are grouped and regulated together in an operon. Most of the mRNA found in bacteria and archea are polycistronic. Dicistronic or bicistronic is the term used to describe an mRNA that encodes only twoproteins.

mRNA Circularization

In eukaryotes it is thought that mRNA molecules form circular structures due to an interaction between the cap binding complex and poly(A)-binding protein. Circularization is thought to promote recycling of ribosomes on the same message leading to efficient translation.

Degradation

Different mRNAs within the same cell have distinct lifetimes (stabilities). In bacterial cells, individual mRNAs can survive from seconds to more than an hour; in mammalian cells, mRNA lifetimes range from several minutes to days. The greater the stability of an mRNA, the more protein may be produced from that mRNA. The limited lifetime of mRNA enables a cell to alter protein synthesis rapidly in response to its changing needs. There are many mechanisms that lead to the destruction of a mRNA, some of which are described below.

Prokaryotic mRNA Degradation

In prokaryotes the lifetime of mRNA is generally much shorter than in eukaryotes. Prokaryotes degrade messages by using a combination of ribonucleases, including endonucleases, 3' exonucleases, and 5' exonucleases. In some instances, small RNA molecules (sRNA) tens to hundreds of nucleotides long can stimulate the degradation of specific mRNAs by base pairing with complementary sequences and facilitating ribonuclease cleavage. It was recently shown that bacteria also have a sort of 5' cap consisting of a triphosphate on the 5' end.Removal of two of the phosphates leaves a 5' monophosphate, causing the message to be destroyed by the endonuclease RNase E.

Eukaryotic mRNA Turnover

Inside eukaryotic cells there is a balance between the processes of translation and mRNA decay. Messages that are being actively translated are bound by ribosomes, the eukaryotic initiation factors eIF-4E and eIF-4G, and poly(A)-binding protein. eIF-4E and eIF-4G block the decapping enzyme (DCP2), and poly(A)-binding protein blocks the exosome complex, protecting the ends of the message. The balance between translation and decay is reflected in the size and abundance of cytoplasmic structures known as P-bodies.

The poly(A) tail of the mRNA is shortened by specialized exonucleases that are targeted to specific messenger RNAs by a combination of cis-regulatory sequences on the RNA and trans-acting

RNA-binding proteins. Poly(A) tail removal is thought to disrupt the circular structure of the message and destabilize the cap binding complex. The message is then subject to degradation by either the exosome complex or the decapping complex. In this way, translationally inactive messages can be destroyed quickly, while active messages remain intact. The mechanism by which translation stops and the message is handed-off to decay complexes is not understood in detail.

AU-rich Element Decay

The presence of AU-rich elements in some mammalian mRNAs tends to destabilize those transcripts through the action of cellular proteins that bind these sequences and stimulate poly(A) tail removal. Loss of the poly(A) tail is thought to promote mRNA degradation by facilitating attack by both the exosome complex and the decapping complex. Rapid mRNA degradation via AU-rich elements is a critical mechanism for preventing the overproduction of potent cytokines such as tumour necrosis factor (TNF) and granulocyte-macrophage colony stimulating factor (GM-CSF). AU-rich elements also regulate the biosynthesis of proto-oncogenic transcription factors like c-Jun and c-Fos.

Nonsense Mediated Decay

Nonsense mediated decay (NMD) is a cellular mechanism of mRNA surveillance that functions to detect nonsense mutations and prevent the expression of truncated or erroneous proteins. Following transcription, precursor mRNA undergoes an assemblage of ribonucleoprotein(RNP) components followed by regulatory pre-mRNA processing.

Large average intron size in eukaryotic cells greatly increases the probability that aberrant mRNA splicing will result in the presence of a nonsense (stop) codon (UAA, UAG, UGA) somewhere within the open reading frame. NMD is triggered by exon junction complexes (EJCs) (components of the assembled RNP) that are deposited during pre-mRNA processing. While EJCs located in an open reading frame upstream of exon-exon junctions may facilitate ribosomal recruitmentprior to displacement by a "pioneer" round of translation, EJCs located downstream of a nonsense codon are not displaced because the ribosome is released from the transcript before reaching it.

These remaining EJCs function as tags for recruitment of UPF1 following the mRNA's transport out of the nucleus and into the cytosol where the RNA is degraded, for example by the exosome complex.

NMD is not only a mechanism for degrading aberrant mRNA, however, as there are numerous examples of normal transcripts whose expression is regulated by this process including the plasticity protein Arc/Arg3.1.

Small Interfering RNA

Small interfering RNA (siRNA), sometimes known as short interfering RNA orsilencing RNA, is a class of double-stranded RNA molecules, 20-25 nucleotides in length, that play a variety of roles in biology. Most notably, siRNA is involved in theRNA interference (RNAi) pathway, where it interferes with the expression of a specific gene. In addition to their role in the RNAi pathway, siRNAs also act in RNAi-related pathways, e.g., as an antiviral mechanism or in shaping the chromatinstructure of a genome; the complexity of these pathways is only now being elucidated.

siRNAs were first discovered by David Baulcombe's group at the Sainsbury Laboratory in Norwich, England, as part of post-transcriptional gene silencing(PTGS) in plants. The group published their findings in *Science* in a paper titled "A species of small antisense RNA in posttranscriptional gene silencing in plants".Shortly thereafter, in 2001, synthetic siRNAs were shown to be able to induce RNAi in mammalian cells by Thomas Tuschl, and colleagues in a paper published in*Nature*. This discovery led to a surge in interest in harnessing RNAi for biomedical research and drug development.

Structure

siRNAs have a well-defined structure: a short (usually 21-nt) double strand RNA (dsRNA) with 2-nt 3' overhangs on either end:

Each strand has a 5' phosphate group and a 3' hydroxyl (-OH) group. This structure is the result of processing by dicer, an enzyme that converts either long dsRNAs or small hairpin RNAs into siRNAs. siRNAs can also be exogenously (artificially) introduced into cells by various transfection methods to bring about the specific knockdown of a gene of interest.

Essentially any gene of which the sequence is known can thus be targeted based on sequence complementarity with an appropriately tailored siRNA. This has made siRNAs an important tool for gene function and drug target validation studies in the post-genomic era.

RNAi Induction using SiRNAs or their Biosynthetic Precursors

Transfection of an exogenous siRNA can be problematic because the gene knockdown effect is only transient, particularly in rapidly dividing cells. One way of overcoming this challenge is to modify the siRNA in such a way as to allow it to be expressed by an appropriate vector, e.g., aplasmid. This is done by the introduction of a loop between the two strands, thus producing a single transcript, which can be processed into a functional siRNA. Such transcription cassettes typically use an RNA polymerase III promoter (e.g., U6 or H1), which usually directs the transcription of small nuclear RNAs (snRNAs) (U6 is involved in gene splicing; H1 is the RNasecomponent of human RNase P). It is assumed (although not known for certain) that the resulting siRNA transcript is then processed by Dicer.

RNA Activation

It has recently been found that dsRNA can also activate gene expression, a mechanism that has been termed "small RNA-induced gene activation" or RNAa. It has been shown that dsRNAs targeting gene promoters induce potent transcriptional activation of associated genes. RNAa was demonstrated in human cells using synthetic dsRNAs, termed "small activating RNAs" (saRNAs). It is currently not known whether RNAa is conserved in other organisms.

Challenges: Avoiding Nonspecific Effects

Because RNAi intersects with a number of other pathways, it is not surprising that on occasion nonspecific effects are triggered by the experimental introduction of an siRNA. When a mammalian cell encounters a double-stranded RNA such as an siRNA, it may mistake it as a viral by-product and mount an immune response. Furthermore, because structurally related microRNAs modulate gene expression largely via incomplete complementarity base pair interactions with a target mRNA, the introduction of an siRNA may cause unintended off-targeting.

Innate Immunity

Introduction of too much siRNA can result in nonspecific events due to activation of innate immune responses. Most evidence to date suggests that this is probably due to activation of the dsRNA sensor PKR, although retinoic acid inducible gene I (RIG-I) may also be involved. The induction of cytokines via toll-like receptor 7 (TLR7) has also been described. One promising method of reducing the nonspecific effects is to convert the siRNA into a microRNA. MicroRNAs occur naturally, and by harnessing this endogenous pathway it should be possible to achieve similar gene knockdown at comparatively low concentrations of resulting siRNAs. This should minimize nonspecific effects.

Off-targeting

Off-targeting is another challenge to the use of siRNAs as a gene knockdown tool. Here, genes with incomplete complementarity are inadvertently downregulated by the siRNA (effectively, the siRNA acts as a miRNA), leading to problems in data interpretation and potential toxicity.

This, however, can be partly addressed by designing appropriate control experiments, and siRNA design algorithms are currently being developed to produce siRNAs free from off-targeting. Genome-wide expression analysis, e.g., by microarray technology, can then be used to verify this and further refine the algorithms. A 2006 paper from the laboratory of Dr. Khvorova implicates 6- or 7-basepair-long stretches from position 2 onward in the siRNA matching with 3'UTR regions in off-targeted genes.

Possible Therapeutic Applications and Challenges

Given the ability to knock down essentially any gene of interest, RNAi via siRNAs has generated a great deal of interest in both basic and applied biology. There are an increasing number of large-scale RNAi screens that are designed to identify the important genes in various biological pathways. Because disease processes also depend on the activity of multiple genes, it is expected that in some situations turning off the activity of a gene with an siRNA could produce a therapeutic benefit.

However, applying RNAi via siRNAs to living animals, especially humans, poses many challenges. Experimentally, siRNAs show different effectiveness in different cell types in a manner as yet poorly understood: some cells respond well to siRNAs and show a robust knockdown, whereas others show no such knockdown (even despite efficient transfection). Phase I results of the first two therapeutic RNAi trials (indicated for age-related macular degeneration, aka AMD) reported at the end of 2005 that siRNAs are well tolerated and have suitable pharmacokinetic properties.

MicroRNA

MicroRNAs (miRNAs) are short ribonucleic acid (RNA) molecules, on average only 22 nucleotides long and are found in all eukaryotic cells. miRNAs are post-transcriptional regulators that bind to complementary sequences on target messenger RNA transcripts (mRNAs), usually resulting in translational repression and gene silencing. The human genome may encode over 1000 miRNAs, which may target about 60% of mammalian genes and are abundant in many human cell types.

miRNAs show very different characteristics between plants and metazoans. In plants the miRNA complementarity to its mRNA target is nearly perfect, with no or few mismatched bases. In metazoans on the other hand miRNA complementarity is far from perfect and one miRNA can target many different sites on the same mRNA or on many different mRNAs.

Another difference is the location of target sites on mRNAs. In metazoans the miRNA target sites are in the three prime untranslated regions (3'UTR) of the mRNA. In plants targets can be located in the 3' UTR but are more often in the coding region itself.MiRNAs are well conserved in eukaryotic organism and are thought to be a vital and evolutionary ancient component of genetic regulation.

The first miRNAs were characterized in the early 1990s, but miRNAs were not recognized as a distinct class of biologic regulators with conserved functions until the early 2000s. Since then, miRNA research has revealed multiple roles in negative regulation (transcript degradation and sequestering, translational suppression) and possible involvement in positive regulation (transcriptional and translational activation). By affecting gene regulation, miRNAs are likely to be involved in most biologic processes. Different sets of expressed miRNAs are found in different cell types and tissues. Aberrant expression of miRNAs has been implicated in numerous disease states, and miRNA-based therapies are under investigation.

History

MicroRNAs were discovered in 1993 by Victor Ambros, Rosalind Lee and Rhonda Feinbaum during a study of the gene *lin-14* in *C. elegans*development. They found that LIN-14 protein abundance was regulated by a short RNA product encoded by the *lin-4* gene. A 61 nucleotide precursor from *lin-4* gene matured to a 22 nucleotide RNA containing sequences partially complementary to multiple sequences in the 3' UTR of the *lin-14* mRNA. This complementarity was sufficient and necessary to inhibit the translation of *lin-14* mRNA into LIN-14 protein. Retrospectively, the *lin-4* small RNA was the first microRNA to be identified, though at the time, it was thought to be a nematode idiosyncrasy. Only in 2000 was a second RNA characterized: let-7, which repressed *lin-41*, *lin-14*, *lin-28*, *lin-42*, and *daf-12* expression during developmental stage transitions in *C. elegans*. let-7 was soon found to be conserved in many species, indicating the existence of a wider phenomenon.

Nomenclature

Under a standard nomenclature system, names are assigned to experimentally confirmed miRNAs before publication of their discovery.The prefix "mir" is followed by a dash and a number, the latter often indicating order of naming. For example, mir-123 was named and likely discovered prior to mir-456.

The uncapitalized "mir-" refers to the pre-miRNA, while a capitalized "miR-" refers to the mature form. miRNAs with nearly identical sequences bar one or two nucleotides are annotated with an additional lower case letter.

For example, miR-123a would be closely related to miR-123b. Pre-miRNAs that lead to 100% identical mature miRNAs but that are located at different places in the genome are indicated with an additional dash-number suffix. For example, the pre-miRNAs hsa-mir-194-1 and hsa-mir-194-2 lead to an identical mature miRNA (hsa-miR-194) but are located in different regions of the genome. Species of origin is designated with a three-letter prefix, e.g., hsa-miR-123 would be from human (*Homo sapiens*) and oar-miR-123 would be a sheep (*Ovis aries*) miRNA.

Other common prefixes include 'v' for viral (miRNA encoded by a viral genome) and 'd' for *Drosophila* miRNA (a fruit fly commonly studied in genetic research). When two mature microRNAs originate from opposite arms of the same pre-miRNA, they are denoted with a -3p or -5p suffix. (In the past, this distinction was also made with 's' (sense) and 'as' (antisense)). When relative expression levels are known, an asterisk following the name indicates an miRNA expressed at low levels relative to the miRNA in the opposite arm of a hairpin. For example, miR-123 and miR-123* would share a pre-miRNA hairpin, but more miR-123 would be found in the cell.

Biogenesis

Most microRNA genes are found in intergenic regions or in anti-sense orientation to genes and contain their own miRNA gene promoter and regulatory units. As much as 40% of miRNA genes may lie in the introns of protein and non-protein coding genes or even in exons. These are usually, though not exclusively, found in a sense orientation and thus usually are regulated together with their host genes.

Other miRNA genes showing a common promoter include the 42-48% of all miRNAs originating from polycistronic units containing 2-7 discrete loops from which mature miRNAs are processed, although this does not necessarily mean the mature miRNAs of a family will be homologous in structure and function. The promoters mentioned have been shown to have some similarities in their motifs to promoters of other genes transcribed by RNA polymerase II such as protein coding genes. The DNA template is not the final word on mature miRNA production: 6% of human miRNAs show RNA editing, the site-specific modification of RNA sequences to yield products different from those encoded by their DNA. This increases the diversity and scope of miRNA action beyond that implicated from the genome alone.

Transcription

miRNA genes are usually transcribed by RNA polymerase II (Pol II). The polymerase often binds to a promoter found near the DNA sequence encoding what will become the hairpin loop of the pre-miRNA. The resulting transcript is capped with a specially-modified nucleotide at the 5' end, polyadenylated with multiple adenosines (a poly(A) tail), and spliced.

The product, called a primary miRNA (pri-miRNA), may be hundreds or thousands of nucleotides in length and contain one or more miRNA stem loops. When a stem loop precursor is found in the 3' UTR, a transcript may serve as a pri-miRNA and a mRNA. RNA polymerase III (Pol III) transcribes some miRNAs, especially those with upstream Alu sequences, transfer RNAs (tRNAs), and mammalian wide interspersed repeat (MWIR) promoter units.

Nuclear Processing

A single pri-miRNA may contain from one to six miRNA precursors. These hairpin loop structures are composed of about 70 nucleotides each. Each hairpin is flanked by sequences necessary for efficient processing.

The double-stranded RNA structure of the hairpins in a pri-miRNA is recognized by a nuclear protein known as DiGeorge Syndrome Critical Region 8 (DGCR8 or "Pasha" in invertebrates), named for its association with DiGeorge Syndrome. DGCR8 associates with the enzyme Drosha, a protein that cuts RNA, to form the "Microprocessor" complex.

In this complex, DGCR8 orients the catalytic RNase III domain of Drosha to liberate hairpins from pri-miRNAs by cleaving RNA about eleven nucleotides from the hairpin base (two helical RNA turns into the stem). The resulting hairpin, known as a pre-miRNA (precursor-miRNA), has a two-nucleotide overhang at its 3' end; it has 3' hydroxyl and 5' phosphate groups.

Pre-miRNAs that are spliced directly out of introns, bypassing the Microprocessor complex, are known as "mirtrons." Originally thought to exist only in *Drosophila* and *C. elegans*, mirtrons have now been found in mammals.

Perhaps as many as 16% of pri-miRNAs may be altered through nuclear RNA editing. Most commonly, enzymes known as adenosine deaminases acting on RNA (ADARs) catalyse adenosine to inosine (A to I) transitions. RNA editing can halt nuclear processing (for example, of pri-miR-142, leading to degradation by the ribonuclease Tudor-SN) and alter downstream processes including cytoplasmic miRNA processing and target specificity (e.g., by changing the seed region of miR-376 in the central nervous system).

Nuclear Export

pre-miRNA hairpins are exported from the nucleus in a process involving the nucleocytoplasmic shuttle Exportin-5. This protein, a member of the *karyopherin* family, recognizes a two-nucleotide overhang left by the RNase III enzyme Drosha at the 3' end of the pre-miRNA hairpin. Exportin-5-mediated transport to the cytoplasm is energy-dependent, using GTP bound to the Ran protein.

Cytoplasmic Processing

In the cytoplasm, the pre-miRNA hairpin is cleaved by the RNase III enzyme Dicer. This endoribonuclease interacts with the 3' end of the hairpin and cuts away the loop joining the 3' and 5' arms, yielding an imperfect miRNA:miRNA* duplex about 22 nucleotides in length.

Overall hairpin length and loop size influence the efficiency of Dicer processing, and the imperfect nature of the miRNA:miRNA* pairing also affects cleavage. Although either strand of the duplex may potentially act as a functional miRNA, only one strand is usually incorporated into the RNA-induced silencing complex (RISC) where the miRNA and its mRNA target interact.

Biogenesis in Plants

miRNA biogenesis in plants differs from metazoan biogenesis mainly in the steps of nuclear processing and export. Instead of being cleaved by two different enzymes, once inside and once outside the nucleus, both cleavages of the plant miRNA is performed by a Dicer homolog, called Dicer-like1 (DL1).

DL1 is only expressed in the nucleus of plant cells, which indicates that both reactions take place inside the nucleus. Before plant miRNA:miRNA* duplexes are transported out of the nucleus its 3' overhangs are methylated by a RNA methyltransferaseprotein called Hua-Enhancer1 (HEN1). The duplex is then transported out of the nucleus to the cytoplasm by a protein called Hasty (HST), an Exportin 5 homolog, where they disassemble and the mature miRNA is incorporated into the RISC.

RNA-induced Silencing Complex

RNA-Induced Silencing Complex, or RISC, is a multiprotein complex that incorporates one strand of a small interfering RNA (siRNA) ormicro RNA (miRNA). RISC uses the siRNA or miRNA as a template for recognizing complementary mRNA. When it finds a complementary strand, it activates RNase and cleaves the RNA. This process is important both in gene regulation by microRNAs and in defence against viral infections, which often use double-stranded RNA as an infectious vector.

Binding

The RISC complex with a bound siRNA recognizes complementary messenger RNA (mRNA) molecules and degrades them, resulting in substantially decreased levels of protein translation and effectively turning off the gene. It is as yet unclear how the activated RISC complex locates the mRNA targets in the cell, though it has been shown that the process can occur in situations outside of ongoing protein translation from mRNA. Endogenously expressed miRNA is usually imperfectly complementary to a large number of nuclear genes and has a modulating effect on these genes' levels of expression via translational repression.

Mode of Silencing

Gene silencing may occur either via mRNA degradation or preventing mRNA from being translated. It has been demonstrated that if there is complete complementation between the miRNA and target mRNA sequence, Ago2 can cleave the mRNA and lead to direct mRNA degradation. Yet, if there isn't complete complementation the silencing is achieved by preventing translation.

miRNA Turnover

Turnover of mature miRNA is needed for rapid changes in miRNA expression profiles. During miRNA maturation in the cytoplasm, uptake by the Argonaute protein is thought to stabilize the guide strand, while the opposite (* or "passenger") strand is preferentially destroyed. In what has been called a "Use it or lose it" strategy, Argonaute may preferentially retain miRNAs with many targets over miRNAs with few or no targets, leading to degradation of the non-targeting molecules.

Decay of mature miRNAs in animals is mediated by the 5′-to-3′ exoribonuclease XRN2, also known as Rat1p. In plants, SDN (small RNA degrading nuclease) family members degrade miRNAs in the opposite (3'-to-5') direction. Similar enzymes are encoded in animal genomes, but their roles have not yet been described. Several miRNA modifications affect miRNA stability. As indicated by work in the model organism *Arabidopsis thaliana* (thale cress), mature plant miRNAs appear to be stabilized by the addition of methyl moieties at the 3' end.

The 2'-O-conjugated methyl groups block the addition of uracil (U) residues by uridyltransferase enzymes, a modification that may be associated with miRNA degradation. However, uridylation may also protect some miRNAs; the consequences of this modification are incompletely understood.

Uridylation of some animal miRNAs has also been reported. Both plant and animal miRNAs may be altered by addition of adenine (A) residues to the 3' end of the miRNA. An extra A added to the end of mammalian miR-122, a liver-enriched miRNA important in Hepatitis C, stabilizes the molecule, and plant miRNAs ending with an adenine residue have slower decay rates.

Cellular Functions

The function of miRNAs appears to be in gene regulation. For that purpose, a miRNA is complementary to a part of one or more messenger RNAs (mRNAs). Animal miRNAs are usually complementary to a site in the 3' UTR whereas plant miRNAs are usually complementary to coding regions of mRNAs. Perfect or near perfect base pairing with the target RNA promotes cleavage of the RNA. This is the primary mode of plant microRNAs.

In animals, microRNAs more often only partially base pair and inhibit protein translation of the target mRNA(this exists in plants as well but is less common). MicroRNAs that are partially complementary to the target can also speed updeadenylation, causing mRNAs to be degraded sooner. For partially complementary microRNA to recognise their targets, the nucleotides 2–7 of the miRNA ('seed region') still have to be perfectly complementary. miRNAs occasionally also causes histone modification andDNA methylation of promoter sites and therefore affecting the expression of targeted genes.

Animal microRNAs target in particular developmental genes. In contrast, genes involved in functions common to all cells, such as gene expression, have very few microRNA target sites and seem to be under selection to avoid targeting by microRNAs.

dsRNA can also activate gene expression, a mechanism that has been termed "small RNA-induced gene activation" or RNAa. dsRNAs targeting gene promoters can induce potent transcriptional activation of associated genes. This was demonstrated in human cells using synthetic dsRNAs termed small activating RNAs (saRNAs), but has also been demonstrated for endogenous microRNA.

Evolution

MicroRNAs are significant phylogenetic markers because of their astonishingly low rate of evolution. Their origin may have permitted the development of morphological innovation, and by making gene expression more specific and 'fine-tunable', permitted the genesis of complex organs and perhaps, ultimately, complex life. Indeed, rapid bursts of morphological innovation are generally associated with a high rate of microRNA accumulation. MicroRNAs originate predominantly by the random formation of hairpins in "non-coding" sections of DNA (i.e. introns or intergene regions), but also by the duplication and modification of existing microRNAs.

The rate of evolution (i.e. nucleotide substitution) in recently-originated microRNAs is comparable to that elsewhere in the non-coding DNA, implying evolution by neutral drift; however, older microRNAs have a much lower rate of change (often less than one substitution per hundred million years), suggesting that once a microRNA gains a function it undergoes extreme purifying selection.

At this point, a microRNA is rarely lost from an animal's genome, although microRNAs which are more recently derived (and thus presumably non-functional) are frequently lost. This makes them a valuable phylogenetic marker, and they are being looked upon as a possible solution to such outstanding phylogenetic problems as the relationships of arthropods. MicroRNAs feature in the genomes of most eukaryotic organisms, from the brown algae to the metazoa. Across all species, in excess of 5000 had been identified by March 2010. Whilst short RNA sequences (50 – hundreds of base pairs) of a broadly comparable function occur in bacteria, bacteria lack true microRNAs.

Experimental Detection and Manipulation of miRNA

MicroRNA expression can be quantified in a two-step polymerase chain reaction process of modified RT-PCR followed by quantitative real-time PCR. Variations of this method achieve absolute or relative quantification. miRNAs can also be hybridized to microarrays, slides or chips with probes to hundreds or thousands of miRNA targets, so that relative levels of miRNAs can be determined in different samples. The activity of an miRNA can be experimentally inhibited using a locked nucleic acid (LNA) oligo, a Morpholino oligo or a 2'-O-methyl RNA oligo. MicroRNA maturation can be inhibited at several points by steric-blocking oligos. The miRNA target site of an mRNA transcript can also be blocked by a steric-blocking oligo. Additionally, a specific miRNA can be silenced by a complementaryantagomir. For the "in situ" detection of miRNA, the use of LNA is currently the only efficient method. The locked conformation of LNA results in enhanced hybridization properties and increases sensitivity and selectivity, making it ideal for detection of short miRNA.

miRNA and Disease

Just as miRNA is involved in the normal functioning of eukaryotic cells, so has dysregulation of miRNA been associated with disease. A manually curated, publicly available database miR2Disease documents known relationships between miRNA dysregulation and human disease.

miRNA and Cancer

Several miRNAs have been found to have links with some types of cancer. A study of mice altered to produce excess c-Myc — a protein with mutated forms implicated in several cancers — shows that miRNA has an effect on the development of cancer. Mice that were engineered to produce a surplus of types of miRNA found in lymphoma cells developed the disease within 50 days and died two weeks later. In contrast, mice without the surplus miRNA lived over 100 days. Leukemia can be caused by the insertion of a viral genome next to the 17-92 array of microRNAs leading to increased expression of this microRNA. Another study found that two types of miRNA inhibit the E2F1 protein, which regulates cell proliferation. miRNA appears to bind to messenger RNA before it can be translated to proteins that switch genes on and off.

By measuring activity among 217 genes encoding miRNA, patterns of gene activity that can distinguish types of cancers can be discerned. miRNA signatures may enable classification of cancer. This will allow doctors to determine the original tissue type which spawned a cancer and to be able to target a treatment course based on the original tissue type. miRNA profiling has already been able to determine whether patients with chronic lymphocytic leukemia had slow growing or aggressive forms of the cancer. Transgenic mice that over-express or lack specific miRNAs have provided insight into the role of small

RNAs in various malignancies. A novel miRNA-profiling based screening assay for the detection of early-stage colorectal cancer has been developed and is currently in clinical trials. Early results showed that blood plasma samples collected from patients with early, resectable (Stage II) colorectal cancer could be distinguished from those of sex- and age-matched healthy volunteers. Sufficient selectivity and specificity could be achieved using small (less than 1 mL) samples of blood. The test has potential to be a cost-effective, non-invasive way to identify at-risk patients who should undergo colonoscopy.

miRNA and Heart Disease

The global role of miRNA function in the heart has been addressed by conditionally inhibiting miRNA maturation in the murine heart, and has revealed that miRNAs play an essential role during its development. miRNA expression profiling studies demonstrate that expression levels of specific miRNAs change in diseased human hearts, pointing to their involvement in cardiomyopathies. Furthermore, studies on specific miRNAs in animal models have identified distinct roles for miRNAs both during heart development and under pathological conditions, including the regulation of key factors important for cardiogenesis, the hypertrophic growth response, and cardiac conductance.

miRNA and the Nervous System

miRNAs appear to regulate the nervous system. Neural miRNAs are involved at various stages of synaptic development, including dendritogenesis (involving miR-132, miR-134 and miR-124), synapse formation and synapse maturation (where miR-134 and miR-138 are thought to be involved). Some studies find altered miRNA expression in schizophrenia.

miRNA and Non-coding RNAs

When the human genome project mapped its first chromosome in 1999, it was predicted the genome would contain over 100,000 protein coding genes. However, only around 20,000 were eventually identified (International Human Genome Sequencing Consortium, 2004). Since then, the advent of bioinformatics approaches combined with genome tiling studies examining the transcriptome, systematic sequencing of full length cDNA libraries, and experimental validation (including the creation of miRNA derived antisense oligonucleotides called antagomirs) have revealed that many transcripts are non protein-coding RNA, including several snoRNAs and miRNAs.

Bibliography

Aaron E.: *Threads of Life: Genetics from Aristotle to DNA*, The Natural History Press, Garden City, New York, 2005.

Alberts B, Johnson A: *Molecular Biology of the Cell*, New York: Garland Science, 2012.

Aldridge, S.: *The Thread of Life: The Story of Genes and Genetic Engineering*. Cambridge:Cambridge University Press, 2016.

Alfred Byrd Graf: *Advances in Plant Physiology*, Rajat Pub, Delhi, 2008.

Altered Fates: *Gene Therapy and the Retooling of Human Life*, W. W. Norton and Company, New York, 2015.

Asimov, Isaac: *How Did We Find Out About Genes?* Walker and Company, New York, 2013.

Bajema, C. J.: *Natural Selection in Human Populations, the Measurement of Ongoing Genetic Evolution in Contemporary Societies*: New York, Wilcy, 2011.

Balkwill, Fran: *DNA Is Here to Stay*, Carolrhoda Books, Inc., Minneapolis, 2013.

Banerjee, S : *Cell Biochemistry*, Dominant Pub, Delhi, 2009.

Barnaby, W.: *Plague Makers: The Secret World of Biological Warfare*. London: Vision Paperbacks, 2009.

Bast, R.C. Jr.: *Cancer Medicine*, Decker, Hamilton, 2000.

Bauer, M. : *Resistance to New Technology: Nuclear Power, Information Technology and Biotechnology*. Cambridge, England: Cambridge University Press, 2015.

Bhatia, A L : *Biochemistry and Endocrinology*, Indus Valley, Delhi, 2012.

Bowler, Peter J.: *The Mendelian Revolution: The Emergence of Hereditarian Concepts in Modern Science and Society*. Baltimore: Johns Hopkins University Press, 2009.

Bradley, W.G.: *Neurology in Clinical Practice*, Butterworth Heinemann, Boston, 2000.

Brookes, Martin: *Get a Grip on Genetics*, Time Life Books, East Sussex, England, 2008.

Carroll SB, Grenier J, Weatherbee SD: *From DNA to Diversity: Molecular*

Genetics and the Evolution of Animal Design. Oxford: Blackwell Publishing, 2009.

Cavalli-Sforza, L.L., P. Menozzi: *The History and Geography of Human Genes.* Princeton: Princeton University Press, 2014.

Crick, F. J.: Life Itself: Its Origin and Nature: New York, Simon and Schuster, 2011.

Curtis, M.: *The Geometry of DNA: A Structural Revision.* London: Blue Gallery, 2006.

Dabholkar, A.R. : *General Plant Breeding*, Concept, Delhi, 2006.

Dando, M.: *Biological Warfare in the 21st Century: Biotechnology and the Proliferation of Biological Weapons.* London: Brassey's, 2014.

Darlington, C. D., and Mather, K.: *The Elements of Genetics*, London, Allen and Unwin, 2009.

Darwin, Charles: *On the Origin of Species* (1st ed.). London: John Murray. 2009.

David M.: *Basic Principles and Calculations in Chemical Engineering*, Prentice-Hall, 2016.

Dawkins, R.: *The Selfish Gene.* Oxford: Oxford University Press, 2006.

DeVita, V.T.: *Cancer: Principles and Practice of Oncology*, Lippincott, Philadelphia, 2005.

Dobzhanshy, T.: *Genetics of the Evolutionary Process*: New York, Columbia University Press, 2010.

Dobzhansky, T.: *Evolution, Genetics and Man*: New York, John Wiley & Sons, 2005.

Fisher, R. A.: *The Genetical Theory of Natural Selection*: Oxford, Claredon Press, 2000.

Fukuyama F.: *Our Posthuman Future: Consequences of the Biotechnology Revolution,* Farrar, Straus and Giroux, NewYork, 2002.

George Kovics: *Progress in Mycology*, Scientific, Delhi, 2010.

Glover, D. M., and Hames, B. D.: *Genes and Embryos*: New York, Oxford University Press, 2009.

Glut, D.F.: *The Frankenstein Legend: A Tribute to Mary Shelley and Boris Karloff.* Metachen, New Jersey: The Scarecrow Press, 2003.

Graziano Pesole; Cecilia Saccone: *Handbook of Comparative Genomics: Principles and Methodology.* New York: Wiley-Liss. 2003.

Groom, M.J., Meffe, G.K. : *Principles of Conservation Biology,* Sunderland, MA: Sinauer Associates, 2006.

Guyton, A.C.; Hall, J.E.: *Textbook of Medical Physiology*, Saunders, Philadelphia, 2006.

Halacy, D.S., Jr.: *Genetic Revolution, Shaping Life for Tomorrow,* Harper & Row, Publishers, New York, 2014.

Hames, B. D.: *Genes and Embryos*, Oxford University Press, New York, 2009.

Hartl D, Jones E: *Genetics: Analysis of Genes and Genomes,* Jones & Bartlett, 2005.

Hartl, Daniel L.: *Basic Genetics*, Jones and Bartlett Publishers, Boston, 2011.

Heider, J. and Rabus, R: *Microbial Biodegradation: Genomics and Molecular Biology*, Caister Academic Press, UK, 2008.

Henig, Robin Marantz: *The Monk in the Garden : The Lost and Found Genius of Gregor Mendel, the Father of Genetics*. Houghton Mifflin, 2000.

Herrero A and Flores E,: *The Cyanobacteria: Molecular Biology, Genomics and Evolution* (1st ed.). Caister Academic Press, 2008.

Jangir, M.L. : *Cell Biology : Fundamentals and Applications*, Agrobios, Delhi, 2009.

Jonoska, N.: *Self-Assembling DNA Graphs, DNA-Based Computers VIII*, Springer-Verlag, Berlin, 2003.

Kallenbach, N.R.: *Molecular Structure: Chemical Reactivity and Biological Activity,* Oxford University Press, Oxford, 2008.

Klotz, J. W.: *Genes, Genesis, and Evolution*: St. Louis, Mo., Concordia Publishing Co., 2010.

Landa, Norbert: *Ingenious Genes Microexplorers*, Barron's, Hauppauge, New York, 2007.

Larsen, P.R.: *Williams Textbook of Endocrinology*, Saunders, Philadelphia, 2003.

Lewis, Ricki: *Human Genetics: Concepts and Applications,* Boston, Mass: McGraw Hill. 2014.

Lewontin, R.C.: *The Doctrine of DNA: Biology as Ideology*. Harmondsworth: Penguin, 2013.

Lindee, M.S. : *The DNA Mystique: The Gene as a Cultural Icon*. New York: W.H. Freeman, 2005.

Luca Cavalli-Sforza, Luigi: *The History and Geography of Human Genes*. Princeton University Press, 2006.

Lumsden C., and E. Wilson: *Genes, Mind and Culture: The Coevolutionary Process*. Cambridge, MA: Harvard University Press, 2011.

Margulis, L.: *Symbiosis in Cell Evolution*. San Francisco: W.H. Freeman, 2011.

Michael R.: Cummings. *Essentials of Genetics*, Prentice Hall, New Jersey, 2006.

Migloni, G.S.: *Dictionary of Plant Genetics and Molecular Biology*, Hawthorne Press, New York, 1998.

Mishra, Shubhrata R. : *Textbook of Mycology*, Discovery Publishing House, Delhi, 2010.

Nelkin, D.: *Selling Science: How the Press Covers Science and Technology. Revised Edition*. New York: W.H. Freeman, 2015.

Prakash, Chandra Prakash : *Cell Physiology*, Discovery, Delhi, 2010.

Purves W, Sadava D, Orians G, Heller C. :*Life: The Science of Biology*, Massachusetts: Sinauer Associates, 2012.

Robin Whyman: *Applied Organometallic Chemistry and Catalysis*, Oxford University Press, Delhi, 2005.

Roobeek, A: *The Biotechnology Revolution?*, Blackwell, Oxford, 2014.

Rorvik, D.M.: *In His Image: The Cloning of a Man*. New York: J.B. Lippincott, 2008.

Sapp, J.: *Evolution by Association: A History of Symbiosis*. Oxford University Press, UK, 2014.

Scriver, C.R.: *The Metabolic and Molecular Basis of Inherited Disease*, McGraw Hill, New York, 2011.

Skal, D.J.: *Screams of Reason: Mad Scientists and Popular Culture*. New York: W.W. Norton, 1998.

Stansfield, W.D.: *A Dictionary of Genetics*, Oxford Univ. Press, New York, 2002.

Steen, R.G.: *DNA and Destiny: Nature and Nurture in Human Behaviour*. New York and London: Plenum Press, 2015.

Sturtevant, Alfred: *History of Genetics*, Harper and Row, New York, 2005.

Stwertka, Eve : *Genetic Engineering*, Franklin Watts, New York, 2012.

Suzuki, D., and Knudtson, P.: *Genethics: The Clash Between the New Genetics and Human Values*: Cambridge, Mass., Harvard University Press, 2011.

Trivedi, P C : *Plant Physiology : Current Trends*, Pointer, Delhi, 2007.

Vasudev Bhatnagar: *Cell Science and Technology*, Campus Books, Delhi, 2009.

Williams, J.G. and R.K. Patient : *Genetic Engineering*. Oxford, England: IRL Press, 2013.

Wilson, E. O., and Lumden, C.: *Genes, Mind, and Culture: The Evolutionary Process*: Cambridge, Mass., Harvard University Press, 2011.

Wilson, I.: *The Blood and The Shroud*. London: Weidenfeld & Nicolson, 1998.

Winston, R.: *The Future of Genetic Manipulation*. London: Phoenix, 2007.

Wright, L.: *Twins: Genes, Environment and the Mystery of Human Identity*. London: Weidenfeld & Nicolson, 2007.

Zhang, Y., S.M. Du and J. Chen: *Supramolecular Stereochemistry*, Kluwer, Dordrecht, 2011.

Index